The Complete *Uncensored* Massage Book

P.C. Anders

Cover image credit: Dominico Gelermo

DEDICATION

To all the massage therapists in the world, and especially those from Southeast Asia, who give more than they get, who make this world a happier and more peaceful place by caring for and loving those they massage; and who, along with their best Western sisters, deserve to be awarded the Nobel Prize for Peace.

CONTENTS

AUTHOR'S DISCLAIMER

This book narrates occasionally true and occasionally fictionalized stories based on some truth, without revealing which is which; the names of places and/or persons have been fictionalized to protect people's identities.

I write as a world citizen, one who has moved beyond racial and national categories: a non-partisan member of the human race. My concerns are humanistic, and my loyalty only to literature, to humanity, to the truth (yes, fiction can sometimes be truer than pedestrian truth), and to my readers.

Also, this book assumes a *male* consumer's viewpoint, because the male viewpoint is the only viewpoint I am qualified to take. A similar book by a woman author writing from a woman's viewpoint is equally necessary, and I would support such a book with all my heart. The word "masseuse" is used inclusively to embrace all women who give massages for a living, whether formally trained or not.

PRELUDE: FOOL BAWDY MASSAGE

In any one of a dozen cities and pleasure zones of Pleasurelandia, which is a region more than a country, you have just to walk down the street, practically any street of any town or city, sometimes just walk outside your hotel or stroll on the beach, and sooner rather than later, you will find yourself having variations of the following conversation:

Want massage, Sir?

No

Bawdy massage.

No!

Hole Bawdy Massage

No!!!

Good for you, Sir. Make happy.

No. [Hey, life is short. No point wasting your exclamation marks.]

Fool Bawdy Massage, Sir. *Fool* Bawdy.

Massage *everything*? [At this point, curiosity, resignation, amusement, and playfulness have overtaken, melted, or atomized your initial feelings of suspicion, cynicism, and irritation.]

Yes, *everything,* Sir!

Include what? [You want to be really sure there's no catch. Besides, you're the sort who likes to know the score.]

Include *Fool* Bawdy. But not include massage ping pong [the male tool].

How about *pong*?

Ok, pong, he responds — pong being the Cambodian word for egg, and also being half the word for balls.

Two pongs, ok?

Ok, two pongs. But *Ping* pong extra.

Not interested. I was just joking, my friend! Ha ha! You want to make my ping pong go ding dong, eh?!

Ha haha, Sir.

Ha haha to you, my friend.

[After a pause, he recovers his poise and coolly asks:] You want *Bawdy to Bawdy* Massage, Sir?

Really?

Bawdy to *Bawdy*, Sir.

Really? Wow!

Yes Sir. Lady take off everything. Nakkid Nakkid, Sir. And massage you with *hole* bawdy. *On your hole bawdy.*

Really?

Velly velly good, Sir.

And ping pong?

Ping pong massage, Sir, afterwards.

Include?

Not include, Sir. Extra. Fool Bawdy include massage with mew. With milk. But not take out your water.

My water?

Yes, your ping pong water.

My water take out extra?!

Yes, sir.

Ok, how much for everything, dammit?

1000 baht, Sir. Make happy happy, Sir. Make ping pong happy, Sir. Sleep velly good. Yes, velly good!

Happy happy, eh? How about happy happy happy? Would that be 500 baht more than just happy happy?

Yes, sir. Too happy. Happy maakmaak.

Include boom boom?

No, Sir. Boom Boom 1000 baht extra.

Why extra? [Of course you know why. You're just being perverse, you're just having fun at his expense.]

You want *massage boom boom*? With beautiful lady, Sir. Have *movie* star.

Hmmm, *movie* star. Let me guess. Is her first name Angelina, by any chance?

No Sir. Angel.

Oh. And has this Angel starred in any movies that I may have seen?

Don't know, Sir. Maybe . . . if you have seen *Thai Angels XXX No.23*.

[Thai Angels! Movie Star! Even a hardened man's resistance has begun to melt.] How much?

1000 baht for beautiful lady.2000 baht for sexy lady.3000 baht for karaoke singer. 4000 baht for movie star. In loom 1000 extra. But no bawdy to bawdy.

Why?

Because bawdy to bawdy lady not same same lady [as] massage boom boom lady. Also extra for karaoke.

Karaoke? What made you think, all of a sudden, that I was looking for a musical evening?

Karaoke, Sir. Lady smoke your banana, Sir! Make *kala-okay* with your banana, Sir. Velly good.Velly healthy, Sir. Sleep velly good.

Oh, I see. And I thank you from the bottom of my heart for being so concerned and solicitous about my sleep, my health, and my general welfare. But let me get this straight: Smoking-hot lady sing karaoke with and smoke my banana, but no light it on fire, right?

Ha ha, yes sir. No worry, Sir, she no barbecue your banana, Sir, no light your fucking ass on fire . . . Sir!

So Karaoke include? (By now, you understand that "karaoke" is their comical slang for fellatio, and you have also picked up a bit of the local "English," or Thinglish, Minglish, or Singlish, in which there are no tenses except the present, and every verb is spoken in the present tense, usually in a subject verb object format, but often dropping the unnecessary part of speech. The Golden Rule being: Never use three words when two will do.)

Ha ha, sir. No, Sir. 500 *extra* for karaoke.

Ok, forget all that. I was just joking. How much for a simple massage? Massage *no* boom boom.

Solly, sir. Massage *no* boom boom *no* have. You want massage no boom boom, you go beauty salon. Closed now, open tomollow molning.

At this point you are likely to be so frustrated that you throw your hands in the air and say, "Okay, just give me everything. And take *all* my money! And take me too! My cherry is still intact."

Because at this moment, your wheels or your chakras are spinning, and that is the worst moment for someone to switch off the power. Because while you may have thought *you* were playing him, the fact is that *he* was playing *you* all along, he has come across a hundred wise guys like you, and there is a 50-50 chance that you will at this point crumble and take whatever is on offer. Because he has subtly sold himself, even if you thought at first you were going to have some fun at that poor local joker's expense. Your mojo wheels are spinning, and now they must either be taken care of, or you won't be able to sleep — or worse, may have to check into the local nuthouse, and you can't let yourself down like that. It's like being in a swank and cavernous but windowless New Delhi restaurant on a summer afternoon when suddenly, there is a power failure, and the air-conditioner stops, and the lights go off.

Many of us will have surrendered at some halfway point in the above dialogue, if not earlier, and be stretched out on a massage table or on a bed, having the wildest time of our lives, sensuality spiced with laughter and total insanity, a scenario we couldn't even have begun to dream of in our home countries. Because once our sexual arousal has proceeded beyond the point of containment by logic and previous experience, we are like lambs led to the slaughter. Helpless and pitiful. At this point, only the physical intervention of Superman can save our souls.

Besides, some of us are here precisely because of this insatiable desire for touch, for laughter, for closeness and intimacy (whether or not we admit it to ourselves), of which the world, including parts of the Western world, has not enough — for even George W. Bush, had he had his pathetic ping pong massaged by a lovely Thai ping pong specialist twice weekly, might never have invaded Iraq and pranced about that aircraft carrier in that obscene flight suit.

On the other hand, who is to say that he wouldn't, in such a case, have invaded Pleasurelandia and transformed it into Texas — or even worse, into a gigantic post-2003 Baghdad?

Ultra Short Glossary for the Otherly but not Udderly Advantaged

Pong: egg or ball/balls, in this piece used with creative license to specifically refer to the quasi-spherical male endowments suspended below the male member.

Bawdy to Bawdy: When a woman massages your entire naked body with her entire naked body, usually oiled or soaped.

Mew: Milk, also meaning "breast" — the word for milk and breast is identical in many Southeast Asian languages. "Big Mew" means "Big Breasts." And "massage with mew" means a massage using the breasts instead of the hands to massage a customer.

Milk: Woman's breast, unless you happen to be in a restaurant; where, if you don't happen to have an infant that you are taking care of, and if you were to order milk, they would most likely burst out laughing, milk being considered unsuitable nourishment for anyone aged above seven.

Water: Joy juice, Essence of Man, semen (which could include semen from a seaman).

THAILAND

Nothing about my years of living in America had prepared me for what I was to discover in Thailand. At first, I would just stop over for 3-4 days on my trips to other countries in Asia, in connection with research for my novels. But after a bad divorce ending in mid-2000, and partly because of Southeast Asia's comparatively low cost of living — a dollar or two for a meal, as little as fifteen dollars a night for an air-conditioned room, and seven dollars for a massage — my objective had now changed to survival, emotional, physical, and financial, until I published a commercially successful book. I started spending long stretches in Thailand and Indonesia, months and months, always planning for just a month or two each time. Unexpectedly, all of these months added up to over three years spent in Thailand and Indonesia combined, and two more years in other Southeast Asian countries. And on these trips, I took my willy along with me. Which, according to one wise guy on the Internet, is one of just two things a man gets to keep after a divorce (frankly, I still don't know which the other one is).

Briefly, I found myself in a scenario I couldn't have imagined in my wildest dreams: totally cut off from children, spouse, home and society. For someone who had lived for years with abundant affection from my wife and children, it was now more important than ever: not just intimacy with a woman, but mouth to mouth kissing. I tongue-kissed anyone who would let me kiss them, sometimes perfect strangers — so long as they unambiguously belonged to the female sex, which can be an illusory distinction in Thailand with its gorgeous and often convincing lady boys, I admit. No doubt it would often lead to sex, but guess what? Western psychiatrists don't tell you this, because they want repeat business from you, and get no business if their patients get cured. But I have conclusively discovered that, for a man, the most effective antidepressant is a loving woman's arms, and her soulful mouth-to-mouth kisses, followed by or interwoven with sex.

At first, after a month's visit to Thailand, when my Thai tourist visa expired, I would return to the U.S. Back in the U.S., I would find myself isolated and in an emotional wasteland, there being only so much fun and comfort to be gained from mocking my own sadness by singing along to Ray Charles's blues, songs such as "Lonely Avenue" or "Drown in My Own Tears", or B.B. King's "Three o'clock Blues." So I began to plot spending more of my time in Southeast Asia, overcoming visa time limits by moving from country to country, and sometimes crossing the border for just a few days, or for 15 minutes, and returning to Thailand.

Then I discovered that massage need not be merely massage, but could be a short cut to intimacy . . . sometimes, nay often, the masseuse was herself someone who had been jilted in love, who had been abandoned by a lover or a spouse after being impregnated or left holding the baby/babies, and who, like me, was also looking for tenderness and affection. And when I sensed that, we were instantly attracted to each other, overflowing with healing love.

This is the unspoken element in all of this narrative, post-2000, the explosive, almost insatiable desire to be intimate with a woman, have my skin brush against hers, and to suck on a lovely breast, whenever I could — some of the most beautiful and tender of the massages that occurred after 2000 would be those in which a woman, usually Southeast Asian, offered me her breast to suck, yes, right in the middle of the massage. Where in the entire boring, fucking New York State Massage law is there a provision for such a thing, and where in the next million years will there ever be one (dream on, you patriots and cheerleaders for the American Way)? I wanted to run as far away from New York State Law as I could, I wanted to be in a land where kindness and tenderness were not regulated, not measured or doled out in coffee spoons, prices regulated and subject naturally to New York State sales or service tax . . .

Whenever the massages spilled over into sex, it would usually be the unplanned result of some combination of chemistry, personal initiative, and excess libido, outside the massage parlor, either in my hotel room if she had paid a house call, or during a date outside the massage parlor and without the permission or knowledge of her employers. Sometimes, it was I who was seduced, and many or nearly all of these women told me later that they usually had sex just once or twice a month, and in rare cases once or twice a week, and were in some cases sex-starved for months, because the local men saw them as "over the hill" — divorced or single mothers. And in every case in which we made love, and a few times when we didn't, I would suck on their breasts, and four out of five times, they would be so affected as to draw my head closer and to close their eyes while I was doing it. Which I found very moving.

But all that happened later. When I first visited Thailand, landing up in the City of Life and Brazen Pleasure, Bangkok, with its signs such as "Darling Turkish Bath," "Pussy Show," and "Sexy Teen Massage," and women visible everywhere, vibrant, standing tall, assertive at times, and often running the city, the shops, everything but the buses, taxis, police stations, and the Army, I was bowled over by how easy and relaxed the Thai masseuses were with the human body, with the body of the complete stranger they were massaging, and what a peaceful and even playful thing a massage in their hands could be. As with this masseuse, Nu: a mother in her thirties. Once I flop face-down and naked onto my rubber-sheeted foam mattress for my oil massage, she draws the blue screen partition around me to shield my nakedness from peeking eyes, and then treats my body as if it were her two-year-old baby's. Her strokes have the fluidity and grace of a champion rowing a boat, the forward and return movements so easily blended into one continuous rolling motion. For part of this massage, she is sitting beside your buttocks, drawing her hands up your inner thighs, and gently giving a feather-soft massage to your gratefully expanding balls before circling around your buttocks and reaching down towards your knees. It is almost as if she had been born to do this. You don't discern the slightest conflict in her as you would in the masseuses of certain other countries, who must ceaselessly battle with an internal tormentor and Puritan censor who harangues them with the suggestion that what they are doing is not respectable, or that certain parts of the body are "dirtier" than others.

And their names! Even listening to the names of the Thai masseuses is enough to make me laugh out loud and relax me. For only in Thailand could you be massaged by a Pook (the sound of a fart), who may have earned her name by farting at the moment of birth. I have also been massaged by Fon (rain), besides Meow (cat), Nok (bird), Mot (ant), Goong (shrimp), Yo, Poom, Boom, and Pooh (crab).

After the first time I entered Thailand, this knowledge of the complete acceptance of my body, this promise of warmth and uncomplicated sexuality, had made such an impression on me that the moment I landed in Bangkok on subsequent occasions and stepped into the taxi to get to my hotel, an indescribable calm and joy would slowly sink into me, making me feel generous towards humankind — optimistic, grateful. And I would think, "What a gracious people. How lucky I am to be here."

Meow and Why Standing Up?

In many a Thai or Southeast Asian massage parlor, any statement such as "Thai massage" or "Body Massage" is simply an opening statement — there are no defined categories, and anything can turn into anything else, all depending on the situation and the mood. Words are just words; they don't prevent Thais from being human and extremely flexible. Especially if something is "standing up."

As with Meow. Meow, long dark hair, short, is called in to my beachside hotel room in the Kamala Beach section of Phuket, an island in the sun surrounded by blue waters and a blue sky adorned by a few powder puff clouds. The hotel's lavish rooms are located in independent bungalows set on a terraced hillside, each bungalow with its own view of the sea, framed by gardens and trees and blue sky. Minutes after I call the receptionist and order an oil massage, Meow arrives at my door with a basket full of scented oils and creams and small towels, smiling, wai-ing, or offering me the traditional Thai folded-hand greeting, her body language signaling an absolute eagerness to please. She's wearing white shorts, and so is her companion, a trainee, an unexpected gift who will also massage me in the process of learning. In hotel rooms, the Thai masseuses, who are usually short, climb on to the usually king-sized bed and in a sense climb over you from various directions, thus becoming an adjunct or extension of your body. Sometimes, they sit on top of your bum or thighs, and sometimes they stand on your body. Admittedly, when they stand on your body, you better protect your balls, or at least pray for them; but the rest of the massage is relaxed and intimate. You rarely encounter the strict separation of roles that you find in Western massages, in which the masseuse is the Director, the Boss, the Doer; whereas you, the customer, are the passive recipient, and you better not make any sudden moves unless you are dying to hear police sirens within the next ten minutes and wish to face charges of molestation or indecent behavior.

Whereas the comely Meow massaged me nude (I was nude, she fully clothed), often nonchalantly brushing over my penis, or letting it nuzzle against her elbows or forearms, warming them and passing on some electrical energy while she was massaging my belly. In other words, the penis was never to her an object of dread, but simply another democratic member of the physical world, like a lamp, or a tree, or a rock, or a pencil, except that this was a thicker pencil covered with skin and topped by a brown-pink hat. There was no need to inconvenience herself or me simply because of a piece of elongated flesh called a penis, an object of variable length (depending on that inner sexual dictator that controls my moods, and is giving me a slight cockstand at this very minute, as if to remind me of its power), no need to get a crick in her neck or a strained muscle because of having to bend or perform a gymnastic maneuver just to avoid touching the Evil Snake. And as her hands roamed freely over my belly, her forearms kept brushing nonchalantly against a now completely vertical cock, resulting in a sudden spray of sticky white fluid into the ecosphere. An embarrassing moment for me, yet she, without a flap, without a heart attack, and without a word, simply picked up a towel from the chair, wiped clean the evidence, and then, with Buddha-like aplomb, continued with her massage. I could have embraced her for that acceptance, for that naturalness, for not putting me on the spot or grilling me like a Grand Inquisitor for that innocent biological accident. Only way towards the end, about half an hour later, when her proximity to my pecker provoked a second cockstand did she ask me if I wanted her to "take care" of it (quite a few Thai women that I have met seem to have this endearing motherly concern about "taking care" of you). Until then, nothing in her demeanor had suggested that she would even honor such an obscene request had it come from me.

Meow, being a little older (perhaps 27), was a bit sedate, lacking the playful sense of humor I found in Pooh, the nineteen-year-old girl with a babydoll haircut who had given me an untraditional (me nude, masseuse in sexy white shorts) Thai massage the previous day, and who was so natural, so much at peace with life, that she just pushed my penis away when it obstructed her lawful path, sometimes watched it in wry amusement, and at other times mock-seriously scolded it as she might a naughty two-year-old boy, *"Why standing up?! Why not go to sleep?!"* Why indeed? An eternal question, standing tall in comparison with "To be, or not to be?" or "What is the meaning of life?" — Pooh's question, even more than the other two, is a question that I have pondered for decades without much enlightenment. At other times, Pooh playfully shook her finger at my erect dick and then took matters into her own hands: she pushed the insensible and recalcitrant thing down to "sleeping" position to make her point. And she was so relaxed as she climbed over me and crossed over me, my big feet and long fingers at times touching, or brushing against, her breasts and her pussy; she was so absorbed in the Zen of giving me a massage, as if her comfort, and my comfort, and the massage itself, were all that mattered, that two separate identities had merged, at least for the duration of this massage. She was no more going to twist her body into unnatural shapes for "modesty's sake" than a cat would, for modesty's sake, lift up its behind and tilt its body so that its balls wouldn't touch and thus possibly contaminate its owner's sofa.

The Hotel Call-In Massage

This is the kind of massage where you respond to one of the phone numbers advertised in the maps, tourist brochures, or "guides", which are full of advertisements whose main interest is to provoke your lust and relieve you of your cash. Many of these numbers offer round-the-clock service, unlike the hotel's own massage staff, if any. This is the kind of massage situation in which anything can happen, and the creative and erotic possibilities are infinite; because, once you are in your room, your privacy is respected, and no sexual practice is illegal in *actuality* in Thailand, the laws to the contrary mainly having been written to please paternalistic Western governments.

One worker that I spoke to, Nan, says she was once called in by a white couple who wanted two female masseuses to massage them simultaneously; the two masseuses were then asked to touch their private parts, and then had them watch the couple make love. She had a big and unattractive pussy, said Nan, and his cock was small. Nan and her friend were embarrassed to watch, but did it for the money. She and her partner have also refused requests for enacting lesbian shows for customers' voyeuristic pleasure, though she's open to a threesome or foursome, especially a threesome, because in a threesome with two girls, it is half the work and double the pay — and one of the two girls usually gets off lightly. Excellent pay for little or no work: that's the dream of the average worker in a tropical country, but especially so in Thailand.

Had the couple called in a pussy ping pong specialist or the performers from a lesbian show, they would probably have had to pay a hefty extra fee, but they would have gotten practically anything they wanted.

No Undie Sit on You Massage

Another widely prevalent Thai technique or trick (depending on your perspective), or massage style, is the "No Undie Sit on You" Massage. The trick, especially used when they are massaging you in your room on the bed, or on a mat or mattress on the floor, is for the masseuse to sit on top of your buttocks while she massages your back. Since most Thai masseuses are small and lightweight, unlike their foreign guests, this is not usually a problem, but an erotic provocation, because if they are lightly clothed, you can feel their warm pussies against your naked buttocks, and this can be very sexy indeed, especially since sometimes, from the pressure, you can sense whether they have pubic hair or none (a mental exercise that can do wonders for your right brain, by the way, and should be a prescribed routine for courses in creative thinking, and Fine Arts degrees at Western universities).

The first time it happened, the masseuse, Goong, had come in wearing a thin jogging suit of sorts, and when she sat on my nude buttocks, her pussy (ooh, my cock protests, I must unzip, I seem to get aroused twice from the same experience, once from doing the thing, and then by writing about it) — yes, her pussy and its surrounding areas rubbing up against my bare posterior through pretty thin clothing (and God, as I write this, a wicked idea pops up in my now Id-ruled brain: that in future, under the penalty of the law, all massages ought to be performed without panties — stop it, stop this nonsense, heck my erection is now at full mast and partly supports my laptop, that is, provides about 2 percent of its lift, now that I am naked from the waist down as a practical measure for writing erotic material). As if this weren't maddeningly erotic enough, the tops of her soft, tender, amazingly flexible feet lay inverted on the backs of my upper thighs and buttocks, with the toes sneakily curving up towards my pelvic fulcrum: any moment now, I thought, a toe of hers could, like some heat-seeking Phantom missile, seek out and tickle my cock and perhaps, as a result, find itself receiving a creamy shower of love.

The other common Southeast Asian massage technique is where the masseuse sits astride you, or allows her pelvis to float a couple of inches above you with her knees on the bed or on the massage table, while she massages your back. When she bends to reach your upper back during her upward movement, her pubis or pussy makes contact with your buttocks: thlap, shlap! As this movement is a circular, repeated movement, the pussy returns again and again to say hello to your buttocks, and if you have any life left in you at all, your erotic arousal is going to be pretty close to exploding point.

A few years later, in a small Southeast Asian town, I was

desperate for a massage, and agreed to be massaged by the only masseuse available at that moment: a Vietnamese woman of around 50, who sat on me in her traditional Vietnamese tight silk pajamas, with no undies underneath. Imagine, a possibly ex-Viet Cong fighter going commando Soon, by purposefully rubbing her thinly veiled vulva against my middle one-third while pretending to be innocent and to be concentrating on the purely therapeutic, she caused a massive and hugely embarrassing erection, which reminded me that sex is all in the mind: the mere thought of the woman's undie-less state and erotic intention was the trigger, and it didn't matter one bit that she was sixty years old.

THE THAI SANDWICH MASSAGE

It should be a universal right enshrined in the UN
Human Rights Charter: that every human being is entitled to
receive at least one sandwich massage during his or her
lifetime.

It was in the back streets of hot, humid, and wild Pattaya,
a former fishing village turned into a pleasure resort for
American G.I.s on an R&R break from Vietnam, now the
sin-sun-and-sea capital of Thailand. It was here, in one of
those massive temples of massage with parking lots as large as
football fields, that I discovered the concept and reality of a
Sandwich massage. At first it was just an item on a menu, an
item whispered to me by some Lucifer-inspired tout on a
Pattaya street ("Sir, Sandwich Massage, Sir?"), but when
eternally curious I began to understand what was being
proposed, I simply started laughing at the sheer lunacy of it,
the sheer extravagant joyous life-affirming absurdity of it! In
the Age of AIDS! Begone, ye fellas! Get outta here, don't
pull my leg! And how in God's name can you protect
yourself against viral invasions during a sandwich massage
unless you were to encase yourself in a body suit —
preferably an impenetrable space suit? And yet, stop and
consider for a moment: what use is an AIDS-free life without

a sandwich massage?

To rewind the story back to its very beginning: One evening some years ago, around the time my marriage was breaking up, I found myself in Pattaya, bored, having repressed myself by sitting in my room for two days with my laptop in front of me, writing. Afraid of AIDS, afraid of leaving my sheltered seaside hotel and venturing into the unknown. For a healthy male to be bored in Pattaya, Sin Capital of Thailand? There must be something seriously wrong with him!

Well, actually, it did help that I had safely ensconced myself far away from the main pleasure zones in a fortress of a hotel called The Ambassador Hotel (which also refers to itself, without irony, as Ambassador City), located in Jomtien, an offshoot of Pattaya and around six kilometers from downtown Pattaya. The hotel fills you with a feeling of stupefaction and wonder: how do they build these gigantic people-cities, where do they get the balls to plan and finance them, and what in hell are these high-rises doing in some quiet corner of Thailand which, only fifteen years back, was a sleepy fishing village in which the only occupation for most men, when they were not fishing, was to scratch their balls?

It is spacious, no doubt: high ceilings, large rooms, an expansive view of sea and mountains and skyscrapers and beach, and of swimming pools so gigantic you could sail a yacht inside them, pools so huge I can see the waves forming in them from up there in my seventeenth-floor room. Coconut palms sway on the beach, providing shade from the white-hot sun. The beach itself is a narrow washout, and may explain the relative emptiness and desolation of this concrete jungle, this insane construction by the greedy and egomaniac financiers that backed it.

The hotel boasts eight massive restaurants, each large enough to house and feed an army battalion; but the total number of souls eating in *all* of these restaurants on this Wednesday evening is . . . Eight! I finally choose the Seafood Restaurant, and an army of waiters and hangers-on waits on .

. . who? On me! Yes me, me and only me, who is no prince, no nobleman, no tycoon, but just a drifter, a rolling stone, an unknown writer! It's a megalomaniac's delight, this absurd turn of events in which an entire restaurant in a 4.5-star mega hotel is awaiting one man's megalomaniac pleasure. And you're not even some president of a republic or some big managing director, but a shiftless vagabond of the Universe, without moorings, without a proper occupation, without a proper income, without anything worthwhile to your name, yet you have the gall to order not a hamburger, not Chicken Fried Rice, but . . . hold your breath, Grilled Plakapong Nicoise. For the simple bloody reason that Grilled Plakapong Nicoise at 80 baht sounds like something you haven't eaten, and is in fact the cheapest dish among the things you haven't eaten (you haven't eaten Minced Pigeon either, but Minced Pigeon is 300 baht). Besides which, the name 'grilled plakapong' has that indefinable ping — well, ping-pong — to it.

And how shall I describe what happened thereafter?

I went into town, see, determined to make up for two nights of senseless, Aunt-Somethingish self-abnegation. I knew that to make up for the asinine sterility and emptiness of the previous two days, there would be a sandwich massage (hereinafter referred to as an SM™), and perhaps even more sinful pleasures, later. The sandwich massage was something whose existence I had only become aware of a few days back from a travel guide, and it seemed like one of those things you ought to try at least once during your lifetime, though I didn't fully understand the details; for though I sometimes pretend to be a Sexpert, that is mostly Talk, and it is by no means a subject whose arcana I have burnt the midnight oil studying (in fact, to be honest — I have no area of specialty or even subspecialty whatsoever, I am the greatest ignoramus who ever wielded a pen or inhabited the earth).

And then, after supper at the fabled Kruathong restaurant, where I opted for the Thai Wild Boar Red Curry, my canines tearing into a few molecules of genuine Thai forest porkers,

porkers who were possibly compulsorily retired Olympian or sumo wrestlers, because the meat was so tough and stringy, I called for dessert to quiet the red chili peppers raging within my surprised, inflamed stomach. Culinary visionary that I was, I chose a house dessert called Green Mango with Fish Sauce, which while quite original if not a lunatic stretch for a dessert, and apparently a rage with ladies according to the head garcon, did nothing for my burning insides. I was already a little high now (the role of beer in this story? Around this time, I was nagged by a neurotic fear that I was slowly becoming an alcoholic, even in the joy that I derived from that one evening beer, and the slight anxiety or absence of joy on the evenings that I abstained), from one small fucking Singha beer plus fucking wild boar, which was actually small wisps of ex-retired-boar flesh Krazy-glued to tougher and nearly inedible wisps of fat, gristle, and blubber, and infused with the Essence of the Hottest Thai Red Chillies. Nevertheless satisfying, comforting to my exotically deprived Nouveau McYankee taste buds. So I topped the Green Mango with a banana (another favorite and symbolic fruit — a symbolic day indeed! — ending, as I type this with a banana split ordered a little past midnight from room service) — a banana purchased from a roadside stand for five baht, thankfully with no fish sauce on it. And then, a short taxi ride later, I walked into that Pleasure Room™ for human bananas, the Sabai Room Massage parlor.

Entering the gigantic building, which from the outside looked like a large theater-cum-arts complex, a smaller, Bauhaus Kennedy Center, I noticed something queer: lots of Chinese or Singaporean-looking males were sitting alone at tables and seemed to be sipping coffee or beer and gazing into the distance, as if at some vision, as if at God descending onto the Sabai Room Massage parlor while perched on top of a cloud. Then, as my eyes adjusted to the dim lighting, I realized that what they were looking at was a human fishbowl, or a glass partition behind which, under colored lights, nearly a hundred girls were seated, arrayed in their resplendent, heavily made up glory, and in pink or blue robes or Thai kimonos, with a plastic number pinned above their left breasts. Far more momentous than God descending on a cloud: a hundred Thai beauties seated on blue-velvet steps behind a glass partition, a few looking bored, but most looking directly at you, smiling, waiting to be chosen and taken.

I am such a rube, such an ancient prude in some things. Indeed, I feel shy and guilty about such things as choosing a woman solely on the basis of her beauty or figure, as if one were selecting a piece of meat without first having talked to it (which would be okay if it really was meat, or else your butcher might think you had gone bananas). Such cosmetically advantaged behavior militates against everything I believe in, and yet, I didn't make the rules, and the glass partition and the language gap prevented communication, so the best I could do was not to choose based on the girl's beauty, but rather for some quality of soul; and not to take too long doing it. After all, I hadn't dreamed of anything more than a sandwich massage, during which I now understood that one girl would be on top of me, and another under me, with me being the turkey in between — and somehow, a massage would be achieved. As I'm no huge aficionado of sandwiches, which I think of as the lazy man's food, it didn't make a lot of sense to me to worry about the composition of the sandwich when all I really wanted was a massage. Anyway, it wasn't a hard decision. It wasn't like I was trying to solve the Middle Eastern problem, it was just a massage of some type, for godsake. So all I decided was to scout for was someone with a smile and who seemed to be in a reasonably good mood, and whose eyes connected with mine. Number 107 had a cute face and shortish hair, and Number 141 had a deepish cleavage. Both seemed infused by an essential combination of sexiness, a peaceful aura, and good humor. (But goodness knows I've not been a great judge of people before this, so let me not fart around as if I made a great and wise decision — it was a pure fluke!)

I chose them, we walked into the room, they stripped and wrapped themselves in towels — these fucking towels always throw me off, why can't people simply and naturally be naked and use the towels only when they need to dry themselves, and to heck with all this modesty shit, we all know what our equipment looks like — or we better.

Anyway, they readied the water and the bubbles and, in a hilarious application of modern technology in this still-ancient-in-some-ways society, a plastic float of the kind fat farts use to float on in swimming pools. And they gave me a towel to cover my modesty — which was a scream, because modesty I have none. I may have a host of other virtues: kindness, generosity, tenderness, intelligence, humor, piety, political acumen, geographical knowledge, soft sensuous hands, mathematical ability, and trigonometrical acumen. But modesty — not an effing shred of it, thank god!

Anyway (there is an eternity of anyways from here to the end), they finally stripped, and they seemed to be softening up.

And then the fun began!

We went into the water and got our uh-uh's wet, and they soaped me while I soaped them. They hadn't asked me for assistance in the soaping department, but as I believed in the proletarian brotherhood of labor, I labored hard to soap their difficult-to-reach (for them) nether regions, especially considering that under the cloak of this humanitarian and philanthropic labor that any NGO could be proud of, my fingers could feel their soft, spongy, and hairless pussy lips . . .

Goodness gracious, the silky smoothness of those pussy lips! What remarkable shaving expertise was at work in producing those two works of art! (I didn't realize, when I wrote this, that certain races, the Chinese and Chinese-related races for example, often produced women who naturally have little or no pubic hair, making shaving and the environmentally unfriendly institution of disposable razors unnecessary.) My admiration for them was high indeed, and like any connoisseur, I bent low to get a better vantage point from which to admire these wonders.

Meanwhile, the women were loosening up, and so were their thighs, their attitudes, their moral and ecological postures, and such admiration was now an eminently feasible thing. And then, after washing each other off (I helped), I lay down, as directed, on the plastic float, and that was when the merriment ascended into a Heaven of invention and ecstasy. I was lying face down on the float, when suddenly I am drowned in the sensation of a soapy woman and her alabaster breasts applying themselves in circles to my back and buttocks, describing arcs of exquisite pleasure and hilarity on them. Atomic particles of indeterminate size and shape comprising my skin, millions of individual nerve endings join in dancing and going berserk with surprise and ecstasy, such is the magic of the combination of soap, water, woman, soapy nipples, and wicked intent.

Suddenly, a pudendum — I mean a prime Thai hairless pussy — goes smack smack smack into my balls (I am totally surprised at the resilience of those usually delicate and tender spheres), as she goes wild with the joy of it. It is as if she's riding a rollercoaster, but her major point of contact is her pelvic fulcrum, that meeting point of perineum, ass, and pussy, which is sliding up and down my legs, thighs and buttocks, and she's reached the point when can't stop herself from coming/going up and down, reminding me of the loony Texan B-52 commander in *Dr. Strangelove or How I Learned to Stop Worrying and Love the Bomb* who mounts a nuclear warhead and sails towards his target like a gleeful cowboy at a rodeo.

Now that I think about it, it's a damn good thing that I had some self-control, and that earlier that morning, the in-house hotel masseuse had milked me and drained me of excess sperm, for it would have been catastrophic, to say the least, had I ejaculated at this particular moment in the History of the Thai Sandwich Massage. My happy flag flew at full mast, proudly. It was a glorious day for my manhood.

At some point in the proceedings, we arrived at the Pure Sandwich Moment. This was when I had two swollen feminine nipples, one slippery smooth Mons, and two silky smooth thighs under my nude body, and two nipples, one quivering vulva, and two smooth thighs on top of me, and the one on top did a fair bit of giddy rolling around.

How can I explain the glorious sensuousness of this? Think of a massage by two women, except that this one used not just the two women's hands, it used their breasts, bellies, thighs, buttocks, and pussies — multiply each of these by two — to give multiple and simultaneous massages at twelve different points of contact, so that, if you were a polymorphously perverse individual (which I nearly am, except that I have zero erogenous feeling in my nails, hair, and kneecaps), inclined to get orgasms from nearly every part of your body, you could theoretically be getting multiple orgasms coming in from every direction simultaneously, causing an orgasmic traffic jam to rival Mexico City at rush hour.

It surprises me now to think that I didn't faint with pleasure, as heroines sometimes do in the more explicit romantic novels as their blond and blue-eyed heroes' rampant "manhood" storms their tender, delicate, and throbbing citadels or Inner Goddesses.

The sandwich was now accomplished. Was it all over?

The girls now washed off the massive quantity of soap and silly bubbles from my body, I helping with the formalities, and somehow, as if we were following a script written in heaven, perhaps by some karmic St. Peter, all three of us drifted towards the bed, where toweled 107 began massaging a partly toweled me.

Whereupon 141 joined us and loosened her towel, at which I gently fondled her breasts, and she was cheerful enough about this new development. Now 107 also loosened up and casually held onto my sky-pointing missile — as if for support while Spaceship Earth was suddenly experiencing turbulence — while she discussed further plans for the evening. Needless to say, with such a weapon in her hand, she had an unassailable advantage over me in any such discussions. For she could easily drive her point home.

Which discussions, it turned out, were pretty thin on abstruse philosophical abstractions and pretty much to the point. Would I like to fuck the two of them? She asked, quite plainly. As if I didn't believe in equal rights and the equality of all women, and would favor one over the other.

At first the price seemed an obstruction — 1,000 baht each, on top of the thousand baht I had already paid at the desk for the sandwich, which I had apparently already consumed and digested by now, if not excreted — but then, my fabled male weakness came into play. Had I been Adam, I might have eaten the apple in Line 2 of Genesis, no serpent or woman necessary, and the story would pretty much be over by Line 3. For 107 still had my cock as a not unwilling prisoner in her hands and was making appreciative remarks about it to 141 (or so it seemed — my laughter had infected all of us and had elevated the general mood), so what chance did I have of resistance?

So it was agreed, and we did it, but what I remember most about this phase of the proceedings was those few seconds when I had two separate fingers in two separate cunts at the same instant of time! Negative charges from one cunt flowing through my positive fingers, through my body and then passing back through another set of fingers into a second negative terminal. The sheer delightful and lunatic decadence of it! It seemed like a finger in the ass of the Absolute and its prescriptions and proscriptions about the man-woman combination!

Happy together! Suddenly, the syrupy old pop song had a meaning! How could it ever have meant just two people! Three is the natural number, the way it was meant to be! If three is a good enough number for the Holy Trinity, it sure is good enough for us unholy mortals.

These were generous girls — they kissed me, kissed and licked my body, licked and sucked my cock. I had to restrain them from overdoing this particular procedure, as I had some vague and innocent idea that this was a somewhat dangerous specialty, considering the number of cocks they had probably already sucked. They also tongued my balls, caressed and fingered my back and bum . . .

These were happy broads!

No doubt the rich are happy, and happier than the poor, I thought (no, I didn't really think it then — I'm thinking it now, while writing this down back in my hotel room . . . so long as we're trying to be honest, let's be really honest, even if it's a silly fart of a truth such as this). Not because, as in Hemingway's famous retort to Scott Fitzgerald, the rich have more money, but because they can afford more sandwiches. More Norwegian salmon sandwiches. More club sandwiches. More caviar sandwiches. More international sandwiches. More *love sandwiches*. And because more women, unable to overcome the basic makeup of their natures (exceptions only prove the rule; and nowadays, on hugely successful television shows like *Who Wants to Marry a Millionaire*, no one even tries to hide what was once not to be spoken aloud), will naturally attempt to get into the pants of the rich and the famous. Though what a burden it must be for these poor rich stiffs to keep their pants on and zipped.

Returning to my two new Thai lovers: the women seemed to know, when we walked out of the massage area and into the lounge, that they had zoomed me up into a stratosphere of ecstasy and fulfillment. I was radiant. How could anyone not see it? It made me feel a smaller man not to acknowledge them as we approached the main hall, not to walk proudly with them hand in hand, but to slink away as if we had been occupying the same space by mere accident, my visit to this huge erotic massage emporium having been in the role of a plumber, accountant, or wall painter perhaps!

I was in the Valley of Death, dying a spiritual death for the past few years, a death decreed by fear. And thou, the AIDS-Scourge of the World — *Great Sex,* which can throw ordinary caution and medical prudence to the winds — yes, Great Sex, which pooh-poohs the AIDS fear-mongers of mankind, has brought me out of it.

At the time I had my first sandwich massage, I wasn't liberated enough, and I still needed to *justify*, to myself, this departure from my normal limits of prudence and adventure. But I told myself: I am a writer. As would also have been the case had I been a gynecologist, looking up women's skirts, fiddling with whatever is inside them, and taking care of their needs is my business.

We writers: we are peephole specialists. With bulging eyes. We bring you life: raw-as-sushi sometimes, with a little Tabasco sauce or masala added at other times, our own particular concoction, never quite what the doctor ordered.

And having experienced a sandwich massage, I have now come to the conclusion that it is, that it must be, a basic human right.

Will the world therefore please provide sandwich massages to its six billion residents? And why not, for god's sake? Surely, a U.N. agency can be created, and a Thai national appointed as Undersecretary for Sandwich Massage? Whereupon he/she can work for the Universal Right of every human being to Life, Liberty, and one Sandwich Massage in every two years.

WILL SHE WILLY? HAPPY ENDINGS & ECSTATIC ENDINGS

On one of my post-divorce visits to Thailand, I had left behind a newly acquired blonde semi-girlfriend, Lucy, 35, in New York. We had known each other rather briefly, but I had confessed to her my addiction to massages. A few days after my arrival in Thailand, Lucy sent me an anxious email expressing her concern: Would the Thai masseuses massage and milk my willy?

I wrote back:

Dear Lucy,

I know you are trying to resolve this awfully important, life and death issue: Will (s)(h)e massage his willie — will he or she?

My answer: No way, Jose, will either he or she; because the owner of the Said Willie is dead set against the massaging of willies, and he has even written a Manifesto on the subject (send $9.99 plus $19.99 shipping and handling to P.O. Box ___ etc. etc.).

True, in Thailand, and many other parts of the world, a section of masseuses, and about one-third of the Thai ones, will, at the psychologically appropriate time, conditions permitting, offer to massage their customers' lingams, digitally or orally, the major reason being that the tip skyrockets from around nothing or 10-20 percent to from 100 to 300 percent. And the reason I refuse is not because I think I can do it myself for no charge at all, and that self-help is the best help, didn't good old Benjamin Franklin say so? etc. etc. No, Dearie, I'm a bit conservative, a bit of a Papist on this (the Pope and I disagree on most subjects, but we would, on this) and believe the Holy Lingam must be preserved for sacred emission only within the soft, wet, and warm confines of the only friend it will ever have: the Sacred Yoni, as Divine Purpose intended it.

Actually, about half the Thai masseuses will respond to your "No, thanks!" with greater respect for you ("Oh, you're a *good* man!" or something to that effect, which is not to say they think the other sorts immoral, but that they are neutral or understanding towards them). Whereas the other half will think of you as a stuckup bastard or Cheap Charlie and either look very disappointed and cast a pall of gloom on the surroundings. Or worse, they will take it out on you by giving you a bad massage in the remaining time available — which is why I will sometimes pretend to delay my decision till the very end, hoping to keep them hoping. But then, the moment they begin to make their move, I try to make my position clear, or else, willy-nilly, I might find my willy in the manipulating hands of the masseuse. And once my willy has deserted to the enemy side (that is, to her side), it may be too late to protest — especially if she demands that I lodge the protest in triplicate.

Also, I don't intentionally patronize the obviously shady places. Shady or not, about one-tenth of Thai masseuses will nevertheless make a sneaky attempt to arouse you so as to change your mind. Still, I'm not a man of weak will power in this matter, and once they know they stand no chance, they give up.

As with a masseuse named Bee (no, *not* half a Bee) at the Regency Hotel. Bee gave me a good professional massage for 45 minutes, and then, at the psychological moment, 15 minutes before the conclusion, she asked, "Want massage for ping pong?" I pretended not to understand, and not just because of the ping pong effect of the tip quadrupling. Though I wanted to ask, just for laughs: "So will you massage my ping until it goes pong, or will you massage my dong until it goes ding?"

I know I could have invoked the Fifth Amendment and avoided answering your question, but I did answer it anyway, simply because it gave me sheer joy to write this email (and I can't say this about a lot of other emails). Indeed, anytime the subject is my willy, I am more than willing to hold forth.

By the way, I don't mean to say I *never* did it. Did it a few times, long ago, out of curiosity — in other words, on a writer's need to know basis — or once or twice out of mere overpowering need. But not recently, because I feel it stands (verb chosen deliberately) no comparison to the Real Thing. The Real Thing with you, for example.

Yours ever, etc. etc. . . .

P

Unfortunately, my romantic connection with the intelligent and sweet but high-strung Lucy — who kissed passionately, for fifteen minutes at a time, and who gave me high marks for my kissing, but left our lovemaking unrated; and whose plans for me included my bringing her *The New York Times* and breakfast every morning to her bed for the rest of her life — didn't last long after that too revealing email (please be advised, all of you men, that while confession may be good for the soul, and especially for the Catholic soul, and chicken soup for the lapsed Catholic soul, it rarely is in a romantic relationship with a woman). Luckily for me though, she was soon replaced by a relaxed and easily risible 25-year-old Thai who had never heard of *The New York Times*.

Until then, though, I had to ward off other Thai masseuses with dishonorable intentions towards my willy. As in Bangkok where, at a new beauty salon near the Phrom Pong Skytrain station, I stumble upon a golden masseuse named Pao, who knows about 50 different ways to massage my bottom, all of them so gloriously tantalizing that I want her massage to go on forever. But she seems like a natural, she simply does it without thinking of it, and if you were to ask her to repeat a particular move the next day, or even to try to repeat it, she would draw a blank.

I am touched by the kindness of her eyes and her soft smile. She is strong, and larger than most Thais, which is probably why she has difficulty finding a sweetheart or a husband, as she says she does. She is 29 and single and says she doesn't want to marry a Thai man because they tend to drink a lot, gamble, and take drugs. (Note that this is her personal prejudice, emanating from a particular class of uneducated, working class women, and one of countless such prejudices and generalizations simply reported without comment or any definite conclusion as to their veracity.)

In so-called traditional (or ancient) Thai massages, which are far less sensuous and far more punishing, and sometimes bordering on the sadistic and bone-crushing, especially if the masseuse is the type who looks like a female wrestler, the primary objective is general body health, to be achieved by means of assisted yoga. But Pao's goal, as is the goal of 80 percent of Thai women who give *oil* massages, is to excite the customer to such intensity that he has no option but to go for the Penile Yogic "Special" — in other words, the "hand release," which is where the big tips come from; or the Oral Yogic Special, or blow job, which is where the biggest tips come from. I don't like specials, I tell Pao frankly. I would rather just fuck.

Like most things in life, however, not all specials are

created equal.

To start with: Hand specials, or the ordinary man's version of happy endings, simply aren't my thing — most of the time. But then, not all hand jobs are created equal, and a spectacular hand job from a woman with soul can be superior to bad and mechanical sex, or middling sex with a condom, because a hand job that involves genuine, and in the best cases, loving contact from soft female hands.

Having expressed my admiration for hand jobs that are a work of art, and that come with soul — they are also, in addition, a good safe sex device, and quick — I have on the whole tried to avoid perhaps 95 percent of all hand job offers. Why?

Because if there is a prospect of good sex in the near future, I would rather preserve my mojo for my sexual encounter. And also that I feel that a man at the conclusion of having been jacked off by a woman looks like a pretty sorry animal, someone without dignity. Seconds after the orgasm, all he's got is a wet tool and a woman with wet fingers who is rushing off to wipe them (if she hasn't already prepared for this occasion with tissues) and to hand him tissues to do his own wiping sometimes. He is at this moment a nonentity, simply a mess who requires cleaning.

I would rather prefer an Ecstatic Ending: real sex, which ends when you come inside a woman, a woman you have helped raise to a plateau of joy, and there's a certain intimacy between you, a bond, a loving feeling, and you usually want to hold her, and she wants to hold you, and respects you and adores you . . . and probably exchanges cuddles and kisses and intimate conversation with you for some time thereafter. This is the opposite of undignified, it is sublime and precious indeed, especially if you hold each other and don't immediately withdraw and rush to the bathroom to wash up. Usually, my post-orgasmic tool shrinks far more slowly when inside a loving, warm woman than if hurriedly pulled out or abandoned and left to the mercy of the elements.

Also, as I come much faster when someone's handling me

digitally, and because, as you grow older, you don't spring back quite so quickly, and this feels like a waste of god-given libido: So many women, so little time — how very true indeed, so why shrink further the potential time that you have to spend with them?

A blow job, on the other hand, from the right kind of woman, with thick, sensuous lips, a great smile, genuine passion, a great head of hair that is loose, lavish, and whose ends are stimulating the entire surroundings while her mouth moves up and down and sideways — such a blow job can be divine. It also helps if your service provider has the right attitude and technique. By attitude, I mean that I have to be convinced that for the woman, what she is doing is natural, pleasurable, and a genuine part of her sensual nature: not something she is doing only for the money. As it happens, I confess have succumbed to a handful (mouthful?) of offers of blow jobs in a massage rooms; but on the whole, I prefer my oral sex to be part of a larger sensual experience that includes plenty of foreplay and real intercourse. A blowjob for the sake of a blowjob — though that is a huge turn-on for the men in the hit television show *South Park* — stopped appealing to me once it was no longer a novelty.

However, as foreplay, a sensual oil massage is unbeatable. A 2-hour oil massage from a sensuous Thai woman is like two hours of high-class foreplay. For me, foreplay, when done right, is by far the best part of making love, or at least equal in intensity and quality to actual intercourse. Imagine getting two hours of foreplay from someone who is going to make love to you? It rarely happens in real life, except for the first couple of years of courtship and sex in a repressed country, and possibly for the first few months in a sexually liberal country. Which is why an oil massage from one of those sexy bombshell Thai masseuses, such as from the Rajadamri Spa in the block on the opposite side of the World Trade Center in Bangkok, is the bargain of a lifetime.

Since then, I have heard of a specialized offering called the tantric lingam massage, which is a far more sophisticated and complete massage than a "hand job" or "happy ending," I would certainly have no objection to getting one every two weeks from a trained professional, though on other days I would prefer to conserve my mojo for the real thing: sublime boom boom.

THAI MASSAGE VARIATIONS

Self-exiled to Thailand in 2001, or rather exiled by dangerous depression and a personal catastrophe, I badly missed my young and heartbreakingly lovely children, and sometimes tried to drown my sorrow, or stuff it to stupefaction, with Bangkok's multifarious culinary offerings, lots of lemon-steamed fresh white snapper, dancing shrimp, and prawn fried rice. At other times, I would seek refuge in the white sands of the island of Koh Samui. Here, massages were my points of connection with the locals, whose language was profoundly strange to me. Indeed, it was only six months after I had made ecstatic love to a lush-haired and buxom young woman named Nam that I learned that "nam" is the Thai word for water — a word I ought to have picked up in my first month. Whereas I only had to walk into a massage shop, and say "massage", and not a word more, and within minutes I would find myself naked or nearly naked and horizontal, having my touch-starved body comforted by the silky fingers and hands of a peaceful, smiling Thai girl.

Sometimes, it wasn't even necessary to say the word "massage". A girl sitting at the door of the shop would smile at you, read your mind, grab your hand, and simply drag you in, while the other girls watched the drama and laughed. And despite your weak protests that you were actually on your way to get lunch, you would find yourself on a massage table or bed surrendering to dictatorially enforced pain relief, pleasure, and heaven. (Heck, it would have been easier to resist the Nazi SS.)

Body Massage vs. Soul Massage

For many years, I was foxed by the signs, in parts of Thailand, advertising "Body Massage." Meaning what? *Body* massage as opposed to *soul* massage? Could one go in for a combo package: some body massage, and some soul massage? And shouldn't any good body massage automatically do some good to your soul?

It was only later that I discovered that the "body massage", often offered by touts with a leer and a wink, was a full frontal type of "body-to-body" massage in which a pneumatic masseuse applied oil onto her naked body, the front of it at least, and then moved her body up and down your nude body in what was a multipronged assault of pleasure: the tool for the application of oil was not her hands, but her entire naked front, with major participation from her breasts. Thus, a "body massage" is roughly one half of a sandwich massage, but without the soap, bubbles, plastic float, and general insanity that accompanies the Sandwich massage. Obviously, the therapists cannot be too thin or underdeveloped, or there would be little pleasure for the man, and not much good for his soul either, unless he were a Calvinist. I would even venture that prominent nipples add at least 25 per cent to the pleasure of a body massage, and that inverted nipples are an immediate disqualification.

The Angel Massage

While the system itself often seems to be designed to squeeze the foreign tourist dry, and to do it with a smile, in the most pleasant manner possible, you can also find a few individuals whose kindness seems to have no motive whatsoever.

Arriving at SuratThani in Central South Thailand on my

way from Hat Yai to Bangkok, meaning to stop for the night at a working class Thai hotel before heading on, and almost too tired to do anything with the rest of the evening, ready to go to sleep in half an hour or so, but tense, I accept a cheap offer for a massage: four dollars up in my room, from a somewhat Chinese-looking, plain-looking woman, perhaps 27, and yet, someone whose expression seemed to show some kindness and attraction towards me. It was in 2002, when the American dollar fetched nearly twice as many Thai baht as it does now, and I thought: with four dollars, what did I have to lose?

When she came up to my room, I, being a German or Swede in my belief in the naturalness of the naked body and in the obstruction to humanity presented by clothes, lay on the bed face down, nude. Without batting an eyelid, she proceeded to massage me. When I turned over, and my erection was now on full display, it elicited a jaguar smile of sorts from her. But other than that, she had achieved a true Buddha-like or bodhisattva-like sense of unity with me; I was not a separate body, but an extension of her body, so she didn't have to ask permission or be embarrassed about touching any part of me. She sat between my legs, totally oblivious to my penis often rubbing against her bare and exposed waist; it was as if her own body part were touching another body part.

Then, it became a little more interesting when once, she simply moved my penis to the other side while saying something, and when I asked her what she was saying, she answered, "*I was talking to it, not to you.*"

Such complete naturalness and spontaneity: it delighted me. For I was to realize that in her mind, the actions that were to follow proceeded less from a calculation of profit than simple kindness, compassion, and love. For when she completed the massage, having observed me yawning in the final twenty minutes, she draped the blanket over me — yes, she tucked me in, like no one else had since my childhood days — gave me a goodnight kiss on my lips like a mother or lover, and left, after locking the door. She hadn't demanded a single baht in tips, as if whatever she had done were a mere duty and a pleasure, and there was no need to stick me up for cash, to produce a long list of needs including kids to be fed, rent to be paid, and mothers awaiting surgery. Oh yes, this is the tail piece, or the tailpiece, take it or leave it: when she had kissed me on the lips and was smilingly heading for the door, I decided to be greedy and ask for a freebie: a kiss on my nipple. (Hey, it never hurts to ask; ask and you shall receive.) She returned to my bed, smiling, and gave me a delicious 20-second wet kiss on my left nipple, and left. Now that was a true Thai angel: bless her and her kind.

The Ah-Soul Massage

Not only do good massages benefit body and soul, but in the right hands, they might also do good to your ah-soul — as an Indonesian woman pronounced the English word arsehole (asshole or butthole, as the Americans call it), or the lowest depression in the valley between your bottom cheeks. This was one of the kickass techniques in the erotic arsenal of Kissanee of Chanthaburi.

Kissanee, who is such a bundle of joy and laughter, and who twice had joyous sex with me, invests her whole body and soul into her massages. She lets her soft oiled fingers graze your bottom line with a feather-light and endearing touch both during the upward movement, which also glazed over the back of the balls, and sometimes the back of your cock, peeping out from between your legs, and once again during the downward movement proceeding from the top of your buttocks. Those strokes are excruciatingly pleasurable, and each time her hand roamed over my bottom line, my cock would shoot out an extra quarter inch, then shrinking likewise until one more stroke made it stretch again.

Ancient Massage vs. Modern Massage

And what about those signs in Eastern countries which talk of "ancient" massage? The definition varies from country to country, but if it is a traditional Thai massage, it generally means you keep your pants or underpants on (or wear the loose pajamas and shirt they provide you), and where possible, bargain to take them off. Whereas with Swedish or Thai oil massage, you take off your pants and everything else right in the beginning, so that nothing comes between you, your 'election' [deliberate misspelling], and the masseuse . . . (though the Westernized or semi-prudish places may cover you with a small towel, to be lifted or reached under when necessary). At which point, the only remaining task is to bargain to have the masseuse take *her* clothes off. (In Thailand, any and every combination is potentially up for sale; for the right price, you could even have an elephant brought into the massage room. For the right price, they will even massage your elephant, or provide you with an elephant that you can take home at the end of the massage.)

The Jaybird Massage

Which brings me to what I call the Jaybird Massage: I kick myself when I think of the five hundred or so massages I have had in the East in which I could have had the masseuse nude during the entire massage for just a few dollars more, but failed to act decisively and early, partly because of my shyness and my fear of rejection. On the rare occasions that I did act, often just ten minutes before the conclusion, emboldened by my arousal or the masseuse's friendliness and perhaps horniness, I would be surprised at how little the woman required to be persuaded to let her skin breathe some oxygen and to have her pussy and ass be released from their confinement within suffocating nylon panties.

The Joint Shower Massage

However in one Bangkok establishment next to the Thong Lo Skytrain station, between shops selling brown roast ducks with defeated expressions on their faces, no bargaining was needed; the masseuse, quite gorgeous with a tall and lovely figure, a woman with the clean and wholesome looks of your sister or your rich cousin, stripped unasked right in the beginning, in all her splendiferous young, tight nudity. It turned out this was a practical measure to join me in the shower, a glass-walled enclosure within the massage room, which was itself a soundproof cabin in the basement obviously designed to muffle the customers' screams of pleasure (or pain, as the case may be). Her purpose was plainly an altruistic one: to help me soap myself all over (and being a gallant and chivalrous chap, I returned the favor), and to also wash herself in the bargain. For Thai women are fabulously clean and will shower at the least excuse, from five to ten times a day, while also despising civilizations where the bath is a rarity. But perhaps her chief design was to make me feel so aroused from being near to and being bumped into by her gloriously naked, soapy body, that I would agree to full sex — which would be a piffling 1500 baht extra. Isn't it amazing how few of us realize that in giving, we shall get, and that generosity is one of the fundamental energizers of the human race?

The Sleeping on Chest Massage

One of the most delightful examples of how relaxed things are in Thailand and Indonesia (and when the masseuse is relaxed, it helps your relaxation; if she is uptight, your muscles clench, no matter how technically proficient her strokes): Once, a Thai masseuse stopped right in the middle of the massage to announce, "I am tired", and leaned her head on my chest affectionately to rest it there for a few minutes. Returning her affection (or else, possibly, I was concerned that she might fall asleep!) — and — I hadn't known her since I met her thirty minutes back — I fondled her hair and massaged her shoulders and back, even as her head rested on my chest. This is how relaxed the relationship can get — boundaries be damned, and lawsuits for "inappropriate behavior" or "sexual harassment" would be laughed out of court and off the front pages of newspapers.

The other massage was a semi-sleeping-on-chest Massage

by a horny 35-year-old masseuse with dishonorable intentions towards me: she wanted me to be her boy friend. She laid her head on my chest, facing my left arm, as she massaged my upper right arm and shoulder. The erotic advantage of that, to me, was that her cheek was in full contact with my left nipple, which made thousands of pleasure neurons scream with joy, while her gorgeously thick head of hair fell over the entire eastern portion of my chest with some strands reaching down towards my groin, like the Icelandic Volcano Cloud spreading over the whole of Western Europe. Such beautiful hair making contact with my naked chest and groin, while I ran my fingers through it in ecstasy: the sensations were indescribable. Naturally I forgave her her horniness, as well as her dishonorable intentions towards me. After all, I am not a man entirely beyond reproach.

The Play With Hair and Tits Massage

Now for the Play With Hair and Tits massage. In NakhonRatchasima, a town that is the gateway to Northeastern Thailand and the region of Isaan, which produces more masseuses per capita than any other comparable region in the world, the masseuse was not only good, she showed her appreciation of me by pulling one or two of my chest hairs playfully. In return, I showed my appreciation of her by placing my hand gently on her breast — at which she gave me the kind of playful "slap on the hand" that you give a two-year-old to tell him he is being naughty. It was done with a smile, almost with the unspoken preface that boys will be boys — and it didn't necessarily mean that she didn't want a repetition, it was just part of the ritual, the dance, which could lead to anything. Indeed, she invited me to return the next day — whereupon she allowed me to lift her blouse and look at her breasts with their large chocolate nipples, which I told her were beautiful. She being 47 years old, in a country where most of the male attention was directed at younger women, my compliment was probably worth a lot more to her than money.

Long before I had started to play with her breasts, I had started to fondle and play with her hair, once removing her hair clip to let her glorious hair fall down her back. After watching me bemusedly for a while, she had replaced the clip, complaining that it was hot. But the next day, she loosened her hair of her own accord just for my benefit. On this occasion, I also played with her curvaceous ass, her soft yet well-sculpted buttocks. That I could do this without even the playful mock punishment of a soft slap: it was one of the great gifts of Thailand and some parts of Southeast Asia, for the ass was the female asset with the least taboo; and it made me glad to be far, far away from "civilization".

The Beach Massage

Sometimes, a massage on a Southeast Asian beach can be a divine experience, despite the risk of, to play on an old joke, getting sand in your Schlitz.

First, because you cannot beat the atmosphere: real blue sky, real sand, real waves lapping or crashing on the beach, fantastic weather. Second, a beach massage is often the cheapest massage available in that country, because the masseuse has hardly any rent or commissions to pay; she can massage you on the beach lounger provided by the establishment, or on a rug, mat, or sheet spread out on the sand.

Recently, I had a beach massage in a country where sex is universally loved but hypocritically required to be kept under wraps. No worries; the plump masseuse had fun playing with me right in the midst of a semi-crowded beach, with people walking by and some seated or sleeping on nearby chairs. Pretending to massage my thighs, she secretly reached in and gave my balls a feather-light massage, and let her finger tips tease all those erotic sub-penile portions, the groin and perineum, occasionally administering feather-light "accidental" touches on the back of my penis.

In a sense, it was an unspoken conspiracy against the Establishment or the Moral Fascist Party, to which she was giving the finger, with my consent and collaboration — or rather, ten soft fingers, joined by one rather swollen finger of mine.

Soon, I had an ejaculation — for which I was unprepared, as I was wearing only my loose and pale fawn boxer shorts — so any semen stains would show as wet spots when I turned over.

Luckily, I had my T-shirt within reach, and I covered my pelvic portions with it as I turned over.

So if it gives you a thrill to risk minor dangers such as these: being caught with a forbidden erection or an emission caused publicly by a woman you are not married to, then remember to pack a dark pair of boxer shorts (the looser the better for the masseuse's hands to sneak in under them), and also to have a t-shirt handy. Remember, you can be arrested for having sex with your own wife in a public park in New York, or even in your own car if it is parked on the road (and some people do it precisely because of the danger of discovery, I know); but I have never heard of anyone in a Southeast Asian country being arrested for a massage such as the one above — or for having a wet spot on his boxer shorts. At worst, they will laugh at him and at the masseuse; and who in turn will join in the laughter. Which is very much in tune with the spirit of countries in which the fish are jumping and the laughter is easy.

INDONESIAN MASSAGE: TRIPLE MASSAGE AND THE MASSAGE-FREE MASSAGE

From the noisy, brassy, sluttish city of Thai angels, Bangkok, I flew into Bali a couple of days after Christmas and settled down in the magical and hypnotic seaside town of Sanur, where I was delighted to discover that it was mango season in the southern hemisphere, and juicy mangoes, sold by big-breasted Balinese hawkers, were selling for a song.

Bali in January is drenched by the downpours of the monsoon, but this hardly dampens the spirits of the Balinese, for whom water is one of their primary elements, filling up pools and fountains, making puddles on the street, and causing the ubiquitous fish to celebrate. In the rainy season, Green Bali is usually greener, and one must watch out for slippery or mossy patches on the hard, hard Balinese stone used on pavements, steps, and courtyards.

Unlike the wild and roaring, tourist-packed Kuta on the west coast, Sanur is a peaceful, idyllic beach town on the south-eastern coast of the island, washed by the gentle waves of the Bali Sea lapping the shore like quiet, understated music. The town itself seems to have come from another century — sculptured houses, walls and gates, exquisitely artistic and lush gardens and courtyards, and temples. This delicate, tasteful town sent me into a contemplative mood: I missed my children, my joyous times with them during Christmases past.

I filled my time walking around and taking in the beauty of the island and its people. And walking up Sanur's main street — a magical street hailing from a lost era, it would sometimes seem — during an afternoon break from the rain, I ran into the Queen's Beauty Clinic in Sanur, Bali.

Here I learned for the first time of the Triple Massage, and my battered and polymorphously hungry soul couldn't resist: because the advertised price for six soft, young, and delightfully ticklish and arousing hands (or thirty fingers) freely running around your body was an irresistible seven dollars, or just slightly above one dollar per hand.

The women had shoulder-length black hair, soft and sensuous, and like most Balinese women, they wore bright red lipstick of a red fuck-me color, and loose, thin blouses in which their breasts breathed easily, and every movement could be observed.

Unlike the Thai sandwich massage, in the usual double or triple massage, there is no soap, no plastic float, and there are no naked women — you're up on a massage table, naked or semi-naked as usual, depending on the establishment's policy. What makes this different from a regular massage is that the professional manpower or womanpower has been doubled or tripled, so that four or six hands are massaging you simultaneously.

I was soon horizontal on a table, my pelvic danger zone fig-leaved with a small towel, while Ketut the owner and her two young employees, Rai and her friend, girls of 18 or 19 wearing thin cotton Balinese sarongs (the Balinese sarong is such a delightful and nakeder-than-naked garment, far more arousing and vulnerable than jeans or saris) . . . yes, the three young women had their soft hands like warm little newborn puppies wriggling up and down my back as if they had been made by their Creator for precisely this purpose. The first session was wild; for while the girls themselves were quite well-behaved, my senses rocked and partied with grossly unearned and undeserved pleasure and sybaritic overstimulation (on the other hand, I didn't deserve some of the other stuff that had happened to me either — so there must be some balancing Providence out there).

The next time, only the two younger girls worked on me. I told them that in the U.S., it was the practice to massage the whole body, including the buttocks. So Rai obliged, so efficiently and sensuously that it had the effect I was hoping it wouldn't — it was lucky that they were so innocent they didn't notice.

Ah, their innocence: these girls seem so innocent in the way they negotiate around my erection and sometimes laugh at it. It is an innocence that is both touching and excruciatingly arousing.

Other than that, what is a double or triple massage like? You don't want to do it too often, only perhaps annually or semi-annually as a novelty and a variation, say in honor of Bill Clinton's birthday or International Women's Day. Though logically one would think that by doubling the workforce, one could halve the time taken, it doesn't quite work that way, and the double trouble saves only ten or fifteen minutes at most, while triple massage is in no way distinguishable in sensation from a double massage except in the elegant beauty of the number three (besides which, if saving time is your life's major passion, why not spend your time more productively by staying home and catching up on the *Encyclopedia Britannica* or planning your hostile takeover of Exxon-Mobil?).

In fact, much of the pleasure of a massage comes from being wholly focused on just one part of your body and noticing how it is being touched, soothed, aroused, the blood flowing into your painful zones and relieving your sore muscles, and sometimes being redirected into zones where the outcome could only be subversive. But this focus gets distracted when two or more different parts of your body are sending you somewhat different nerve-stimulation messages at the same time. Because no two pairs of hands or touches can ever be the same, every masseuse having her unique fingerprint or touchprint, so to speak; as a result, as if by some weird mathematical formula, the two or three different sources of pleasure or therapeutic stimulation nearly cancel each other out.

And yet you can't help feeling a certain wonder, a certain sense of awe and regal, luxurious satisfaction at being so indulged in and pleasured by two young women, their four soft hands serving you and only you. It's partly an intellectual thrill to realize that you, poor sod, who has been so touch-starved in the West, is suddenly being showered with attention and digital love by two nubile females. It is as divine as a special blessing from the Dalai Lama, a rare sensation comparable to what a California group called the Human Awareness Institute describes as a Shower of Love, in which half a dozen people touch you and feel you with their hands at the same time. While the therapeutic reduction of pain and increased circulation also happens in a Double or Triple Massage, it happens as a side-benefit of so much movement and manipulation, and is not the chief focus of it. Because I believe that the therapeutic reduction of pain occurs through consciousness: first the focus on the pain, then on its release, and then on the absence of pain. And when six lovely hands are running like hyperactive bunnies up and down your nude body, pain relief is not likely to be the top item on your list of priorities.

The Nyoman Massage

If you've visited Bali, there is a 25 percent chance you have received the Nyoman massage, but never realized it, because nearly one-fourth of all Balinese men and women are named Nyoman (or Koman), meaning they happen to be the third child of their parents. Twenty days after my arrival in Bali, I find myself in Candidasa, a quiet beach and temple town northeast of Sanur on Bali's east coast, painted boats with blue sails in the distance, with the occasional lean boatman rowing a Buddha-fat Western tourist; and a rocky island on the southeastern horizon lazing under a veil of mist, while Bali's presiding sacred mountain Gunung Agung rises majestically through the clouds on a clear morning on the Western horizon, its calm façade belying its hot volcanic interior, quiet for now, but far from dead. It is a sunny late morning, and I'm already feeling horny thinking of my impending massage with Nyoman, who met me earlier this morning and held both my hands in hers for a long, long time, as if she were meeting a long-lost beloved or friend (such an unexpected gift of love and intimacy that it raised my erotic temperature by about 100 degrees, which was the last thing I needed at that point, when I was already at boiling temperature — but heck, who's going to refuse a gift?).

Also, she asked me if I was sendiri, or traveling alone — when an Indonesian woman asks a man that question, it usually means that she has designs on him. Well, so what, I think at that moment, my penis doing most of the thinking for me. Damn it: massages are all about sex, and why not? Life is short! Fuck it, even if it has taken me eighteen years into my massage obsession to learn this.

And yet: wait a moment. Nothing is *all* about sex! Even sex is not all about sex. Sex is about a program of the species, and it's about connection with another human being, the search for a soul mate, for excitement and life. Every time I honor sex, I honor the Goddess Venus (or the Yoni Goddess, if you will). So to all the idiots in my lives past who have ever said to me, "You *only* think about sex," I now issue a resounding "Boo!" to their microscopic, tight-assed brains! They lack understanding, and they insult the Cosmic Yoni that created them.

Other variations offered by Bali's glorious spas include the mandi lulur massage, which is an exfoliating and body polishing massage using a paste of sandalwood, turmeric, groundnuts, rice, and other scented woods, followed by a hot shower and the application of a yoghurt mix; and massages in which, for part of the time, your body is scrubbed with milk or immersed in a tub full of rose petals, often by female staff who are Javanese, not Balinese (I have invariably found Javanese women, including the Madurese, to be among the world's sexiest, far outshining most of their island neighbors including, sorry, the Balinese). Cheap by Western standards, some of these massages can be quite expensive by Indonesian standards, and I myself nearly always chose the cheapest no-frills massage joints, where if the masseuse went well beyond the call of duty, I felt the indescribable emotional satisfaction of knowing that I had been the beneficiary of her generosity and sexuality, the beauty of her personality, and the beginnings of that warm feeling called love — and that my tiny payment had nothing to do with it. This realization was as much of a turn-on as the massage itself.

* * * *

When I was first introduced to the massage system in Jakarta, as I understood it, it blew more than my mind: I went in a lion and came out like a lamb.

Unlike mainly Hindu Bali, a temple-rich island and culture unto itself, and where a vast superstructure of tourism and tourist facilities coddles the newbie tourist and results in an island overrun in pockets by Western tourists, exploitative touts, and tourist service industries, Jakarta in the mainly Muslim island of Java exists mainly for itself, for its own citizens, for the millions from different social classes who form its citizenry, and it has no time to pander to tourists. Even if armed with a map and a guide, a tourist can feel quite lost in the Big Mango (as the city is affectionately called), for it is hard, in some sections of the city, to find a single person who speaks or is willing to speak English.

Visiting Jakarta for the first time after my second trip to Bali in March 2001, it was as if I had landed in a new world. And in this hot tropical city of phallic skyscrapers, flat grey slums, and broad streets through which rivers of humanity flow — except during flood-prone spells in the rainy season when the sky is permanently grey — I discovered some of the most touching, endearing, and fascinating human beings. As indeed I did in other parts of Java, an island with endless and awe-inspiring volcanoes.

Soon after my arrival, I urgently needed a massage, as I do after all long journeys to a new country: the stress of packing, dashing off to the airport, immigration, security, and customs, long confinements within congested airplanes, and the lifting of heavy suitcases. So after checking into my hotel in old North Jakarta, a mix of residential and commercial, with not a white face around, I started following my nose, looking for a massage place. The word for massage in the Indonesian language is pijat — a simple five-letter word, like the word for love (cinta). As Indonesia uses the Roman script for its language, it is easy for a foreigner to spot the signs; walking the streets around my hotel, I noticed plenty of signboards for pijat, boards announcing the names of the establishments: Pijat Meksiko, Pijat Intan, Pijat Berlian (how health-conscious the Indonesians must be, I thought).

And walking in, I discovered that the system was pretty simple. You enter a modest reception room, where a receptionist and a couple of lackeys, usually all women, are hanging around relaxed, chatting (it makes a huge difference when a massage joint is run by women — so much more affectionate, relaxed, and non-threatening). They stop chatting to point out a gallery of photographs of luscious-looking women pasted under a sheet of glass on the receptionist's desk. Below each photograph, there is a name: Yuni, Linda, Ati, and so on, simple and endearing Indonesian girl names, and a color (green for available, red for busy or not available). Once you've chosen the photograph of the masseuse of your preference, the system is simple: You fuck the young ones, the ones between 19 and 25-26 years old (in the latter bracket, only the women who have remained slim and pretty); or you get massaged by the older ones, who are between 28 and 38. That's the general rule, but you do have some choice: you can fuck the older ones if you insist (they'll be grateful, and they may even be far more proficient in lovemaking, not to speak of the Sixty-Four Arts), but don't ever, ever expect to get a massage from the young ones.

At least this is the way I was accidentally introduced to massage and fucking in Jakarta. Entering one of the places advertising massage, I had asked for a massage, and was asked to choose a masseuse from the photographs. "Her," I said, pointing to a delightful girl, who was actually present in the flesh, in the reception area, and who turned out to be Inggit.

"She is not available for massage, only for fucking," replied the slightly offended, slightly amused boss or chief receptionist, looking at me like I must be some weird hick not to know the difference.

I remember thinking: what a difference between two countries inhabited by brown people, using languages with deep Sanskrit roots, culturally connected in other ways, and separated by a mere two thousand miles of ocean: India and Indonesia.

Consider: in India, you could get thrown out of the building, and perhaps even packed off to jail, for merely *asking* for a fuck — unless you were an Indian film director auditioning for the female cast. In Indonesia, fuckers, regardless of their class or worldly position, are welcomed with open arms, given the red carpet treatment, and treated as if they were exercising their birth right. Not only that, if you are a massage-only seeker, and point to the wrong woman and ask for a massage instead of a fuck, you not only insult the woman (who is higher in the caste system of such establishments), you insult the establishment, establish yourself to be a weirdo, and get perilously close to being thrown out on your ear.

Yes, while fuckers are welcomed like heroes, with broad smiles, men who ask for pure massages are looked at slightly suspiciously and warily, if not scornfully. Because, of course, if you go *only* for a massage, that could mean only one thing: you are too old, impotent, lack "power," and so are beneath pity or even contempt. ("Power" or potency is such an important goal or obsession in Indonesia, next in importance only to the Presidency, that you will find hundreds of shops openly selling "obatkuat" or medicines for sexual power — aphrodisiacs, in other words.) Massage for massage's sake, in the opinion of these people, is something engaged in by women, weaklings, and effeminate or older men, whereas real men spend their time drinking, gambling, making money, and fucking.

What I didn't know at the time, and it took me a few more trips and visits to different parts of Jakarta to discover this — was that the modestly priced hotel I had chosen was located in a red light area the size of a medium-sized city. Which was an easy mistake for a newcomer to make, because Jakarta has massive but not exclusive red light zones in which hundreds of normal families also carry on their normal middle class lives unperturbed and almost indifferent to what's going on in the very next lane. In other parts of Jakarta, I would later notice signs for "Pijat Refleksi" — which meant reflexology massage, or some combination of Shiatsu and Javanese massage, mostly with underwear on or under a sheet minus undies. There was no fucking going on in there, at least not on a regular basis. I also finally discovered regular spas offering oil massage; the booths were separated by thin screens, and the only hanky panky possible was a hand job camouflaged by a towel — but no fucking whatsoever.

Of course, in the above paragraphs, I am speaking of Java, and particularly of old, traditional Jakarta — not its Western expat pockets or Bali, where pure massages are abundant, the culture having reinvented itself partly to serve well-off Western tourists. In such Westernized pockets, massages run a wide gamut from the sandy massages given by steel-fingered, hardy peasant women on Kuta Beach for as little as three dollars an hour to the sophisticated massages in joints smelling of flowers and incense where beautiful young women fit to be king's consorts massage you for eight dollars an hour and above).

However, it is a general rule that in countries like Thailand

and Indonesia, if a relatively healthy man asks a taxi driver to take him to a massage place, the taxi driver will nearly always take him to the shady places — not just because of the near certainty of his getting a commission from the joint itself, but also because of the general assumption that if you are reasonably healthy male between 18 and 50 years of age, your overwhelming need is to get fucked (or perhaps they can read the urgency in your face, and read exactly how much in need of a good fuck you are). Double that conviction for foreign males, who are believed to be either constitutionally hornier than locals, or sex-starved . . . or both. I don't wish to pretend that I was above fucking — after all, these were the years just after my very painful divorce, and I was pretty virile at the time, and tried to soothe my emotional pain and emptiness with both real massages as well as loads of fucking, often from women who were pretty horny themselves and always appreciated a good lover, a lover who filled them and took care of their entire bodies instead of coming and going in a heaving rush.

Besides, words are simply representations of meanings or concepts, and in different contexts and cultures, they represent different concepts. Over the years, traveling in various countries, I have realized that a massage is not supposed to mean, necessarily, a massage, but often is a euphemism for a broader range of services. Indeed, even after I picked up some of the local language, I would be frustrated in my attempts to obtain a decent massage at some massage joints in the red light area, though I did end up getting an enormously probing massage at a few. Sometimes, hurting badly, and unable to find an obviously purely massage joint, I would show up at the dubious massage place and plead, "I want *only* a massage please." They would assign you a woman, for they don't want to turn away your business, being not that busy or rich most of the time. But then, the assigned masseuse resents you for not asking for more; she keeps inciting you to change your mind, hoping to earn the higher fee for the non-massage services.

And today, nearly one year after I came to understand the system, I still fell into the same trap: going to a place looking for a serious massage — because sometimes, the pain is the primary feeling, and the erotic need is not the pressing issue in your mind — but ending up getting fucked. What can I say? I'm only human. Where else in the world could you get fucked as easily as you do in Jakarta? And why should I or any of us put on that highbrow hypocrisy and pretend that we are too good, noble, or high-minded for a mere pedestrian fuck with a lovely, long-haired, and affectionate young Indonesian woman? As the Monty Python song goes, "Always look on the bright side of life [whistle whistle whistle]."

Briefly, how did my pure purpose of massage get diverted into a fuck this one time? Because the woman, perhaps 29 (and because of her having crossed the age of 25, a dedicated masseuse), left me so horny, my whole body, every muscle in it, was quivering like jelly, begging to be satisfied. I describe it in contemporaneous words: "The woman is so completely natural and earthy she is nondiscriminatory about parts of my body; she doesn't draw an invisible line around the anus and such-like spots beyond which she won't massage; indeed, she massages the line itself, the crack."

What I also found indescribably erotic and touching, because it seemed such an unconscious and natural gesture, was the way she rested her oil bottle, which was a bit cool, on the back of my balls and on my anus; which made perfect sense, because in that position it was unlikely to topple over. Indeed, it was so well propped up that it might, in case of an earthquake, have retained its position even though the walls around it crumbled. Later, lacking a saucer, she poured a bit of cream into the slight depression on my lower back just above my buttocks. She then applied that cream to the rest of my body, gently, slowly, in circular motions, with the tips of her fingers and the feather-light brushes from her nails. After about twenty minutes of this, I was so helpless with lust that I would have willingly fucked a sheep. Luckily I didn't have to, for when she noticed my tool pointing at the sky, and could read the begging expression on my face, she needed no words, did not bargain, asked for nothing at all: wordlessly, she just took off her clothes in one quick movement and mounted me. (And yes, Your Honor: I did not resist, fearing that resistance would be futile.)

THE MASTER WHO BECAME A SLAVE

If I wasn't cheap (or, if you are inclined to be kinder to me, and truthful besides: if I wasn't racked by the endless financial anxiety of a homeless wanderer though not yet a penniless man, and one who has never in his entire life owned a square inch of property, or even a time share that pretends to be property); if I wasn't always trying to shave a few bucks, or even a single buck, off the massages I seemed to endlessly need, of which my pain-wracked, touch-hungry, woman-loving body is an endless slave, I would never have met Inul the Good, Inul the Great Soul, Inul the Happy Slave. Thank you, oh God, for giving me this unfortunate, often distressing and debilitating trait, for it was the reason Inul entered my life.

Jakarta, the steamy capital of a magnificent country, a capital city filled with more horny women than populate some entire countries, a city whose temperature never goes below 23 degrees and almost always hovers between 28 and 35 degrees Centigrade: tropical heat that the thin skin of the average male's balls is powerless to resist, and that probably steams up the women's cunts too.

I have by now spent a month in Jakarta, usually living in 3.5-star hotels, which at this time in 2002, on account of the weakness of the local currency (around 12,000 rupiah to the dollar, which can fetch you a pretty nice local meal), are pretty cheap, twenty-five to thirty-five dollars a night for a large and lush bed in a large room with large window, ice-cold airconditioning, a pool, and a nice desk for writing, yes writing, which is the only way I can justify my trips and indeed, my presently dubious existence. And what I have overspent on hotel rooms, I save by eating common-man Indonesian food, like Nasi Campur and Nasi Goreng, and curried meals like sapi rendang (spicy beef in thick gravy) with rice or Ikan Kare — a thick yellow fish curry — in Masakan Padang restaurants that cost between one and two dollars. And one day, I am passing by this pijat or massage place in the dirty, old part of the city, North Jakarta, near a shopping-entertainment complex called Taman Anggrek, when a sign advertising a massage for about two dollars an hour grabs me. Two dollars an hour in Jakarta! How could I miss that? At this point in my suddenly lonely life, I would pay two dollars an hour simply to be in the same room with a woman and have her just shake my hands and treat me like a human being. So I dash up the rickety wooden stairs, and tell the waiting masseuses right away that I am going to need no sex, only massage, is that clear? And they say, ""Fine, fine, we understand, okay, walk this way Sir, the masseuse will be with you in a minute."

A thin, short, and shorthaired girl named Inul who comes from East Java near Bali followed me into my cubicle, and I made the mistake of taking off my shorts and climbing onto the table in my tiny but loose boxer shorts, so she could better reach remote portions of my back. Heck, why just my back, she could reach practically anything she had a mind to reach.

Rabbit eyes and swollen lips, a musical laugh, and an irrepressible spirit: that's what Inul had. Anyway, suddenly, Inul's hands caressed my bum crack in a most intimate way. And I am so moved, so transported, to think that his woman, who hadn't known of my existence in the last million years, and not until ten minutes ago, was so intimate, so friendly, so loving . . . and that, on top of all this, she would call me "Master," again and again.

It doesn't really matter now whether her use of the word Master was a result of misunderstanding English, in which she had a vocabulary of around 15 random words. Whatever the cause, the "Master" itself was worth the entire price of the massage. How even the most democratic, anti-authoritarian, and anti-slavery among us secretly yearn to be masters, how we are tired of being enslaved by rules, by the System, by the labyrinthine requirements of political correctness, and by the various colonizing officers of the law, of literature, and of publishing. A woman who calls you "Master" has you in her pocket. Paradoxically, in calling you Master, she has *enslaved* you. "Sir" is nothing. Even a police officer who is just about to arrest you may call you "Sir", and in such cases the "Sir" is almost Sir-castic.

But "Master"? That has cachet. It has substance and weight. In these increasingly and depressingly democratic times, one would willingly journey ten thousand miles to the deepest jungle to hear this sweet word.

"Don't press so hard over here, okay?"

"*Okay, Master.*"

I almost want to stop my narration right at this point, because back in my room later, where I am writing this naked (a clothes-enslaved man never lets slip an opportunity to be naked with impunity), I notice my foreskin gently retracting as my cock starts to expand at the thought of what happened: regardless of how little it was.

She talked endlessly, nearly all of it in Indonesian, and though I was charmed by the sound of her voice and her talking to me as if to an old, old friend, and delighted by how much Indonesian I could manage to understand, I once had to ask her to be silent for a little while, just so I could concentrate on the pleasure of the massage. Then, she said something about my chest being hairy, and how little body hair she had, even under her arms (and she lifted her armpits to show me).

"How about there?" I asked, pointing to her pussy.

"Very little hair there," she said.

"Can I see?" I said, not at all expecting to be taken seriously, prepared even to hear an outraged response. If one is an enquiring writer, these are the risks one must take.

To my surprise, within seconds, she was unbuttoning her pants as if it were the most natural thing in the world and pulled them down to show her small, girl-like pussy. It was a sweet pussy in its own way, and almost made me doubt that she really had had a baby, as she claimed.

A little later, I asked her for a kiss and tongued her. She withdrew my kissing privileges after a very short while, pointing to her pussy and expressing her frustration, as if to say, "No, your kissing is making me too hot. Give me that!"— pointing at my cock, which I had protectively hidden from her view with the help of my boxer shorts. She begged and begged until I allowed her to see more and then nearly all of my cock. That's all I allowed her to do on that first occasion: to see it and touch it briefly. Then I ordered her, my new little brown slave, to return to the massage. (I only use the word slave post-facto, post-coitally, and ironically in my typical fashion of literary excess, and indeed many years later while reliving the event as an analytical writer, a pseudo-pointy-headed pseudo-intellectual; at the time I regarded her with nothing other than love, excitement, and gratitude for her touch, her warmth, her humanity.)

It was only on my second visit, the following day, surprisingly (for it seems to go against the natural order things, which usually progress lower, not upward), that I was blessed with a vision of her tits.

One of the most erotic things about the Indonesian language, which is a comment on the culture itself, is that the word for "milk" — susu — and the word for "breast" are one and the same. So you can ask a woman for milk, and she could lift up her blouse and un-pop her breasts, and that would be a perfectly legitimate response (a few times, indeed, even when they *know* you mean the white liquid that is squeezed out of a cow's teats, they will, just as a joke, lift up their blouses — anything worth a laugh is too precious to pass by, and even more so for bored Thai bargirls, the Thai word for milk, nom, also being identical to the word for breast.). Indeed, so legitimate and wholesome — as legitimate and wholesome as a glass of milk in dairy-besotted America — are tits in Indonesia that until only about fifty years back, much of Indonesia was a topless country. You still find that certain stubborn old women in the rural areas of Bali follow a born-free, stay-free, "Keep your bloody blouses off my sacred tits" policy regarding their breasts. And how relaxed the women are with them. To see a Balinese woman nursing her baby is one of the most glorious, most life-affirming, most inspiring sights in the world. Almost none, whether high or low, tries to hide her nipple, and thus suffocate the baby with excessive covering, denying it the full grasp, tactile pleasure, and warmth of her bosom, or the sound of her throbbing heart. None will allow the gaze of a stranger to cause her to deny her baby the sovereign right of a god, a dewata, which is what a young Balinese is. Sometimes the blouse is fully lifted to expose both breasts, even though the baby can obviously handle just one at a time.

But I was with Inul in neighboring Java — almost the same island culture and attitudes, though unlike Hindu Bali, Java was predominantly Muslim, as was Inul. And so natural was my Inul, the Javanese girl who was massaging me, a girl with a short bob cut (not a turn on for me personally, I like my romantic partners' hair a bit longer), that when I asked her if I could see her breasts, they popped out with no trouble or hesitation, and then, for a while, while I cupped and fondled her breasts, recharging the batteries of my depleted, divorced, and atomized soul with this human contact from someone who was more whole, had more love and kindness (besides milk in the Indonesian sense) to offer than a hundred New York State law-abiding masseuses. Indeed, she kept on talking to me as if nothing, nothing at all was happening. I mean, there wasn't the slightest inflection in the conversation to show that hers was a guy's-hands-on-a-woman's-tits speech. Surprising, because I was also acquainted some time earlier with another Javanese woman who sometimes shuddered and had an orgasm at the very touch of my hands on her bare nipples.

Inul's tits were no great shakes, of course — not istimewa or special but biasa or ordinary, though I love them all, all tits great and small, pointy and inverted (though I have a special weakness for tits with large areolas and swollen nipples), tiny as well as udderly abled udder wonders: God bless em all, the entire universe of tits that the Goddess in Her Infinite Mercy occasionally gifts to us otherwise wretched men — but that's not the point. The point was that to *her*, breasts were natural, and the bra and blouse were simply an encumbrance she was glad to be free of for about five minutes. Finally, the distraction was too great for me, the refugee from "civilization" who had too long been its prisoner. I didn't want an erection, and though for other reasons I already had an erection, I didn't want to harden it further by having her tits within tempting reach, because that was not what the doctor ordered, that would not help my wounded, love-bitten cock on the road to recovery. So guess what I did? You wouldn't in a million years believe what happened, but it really did: yes I, World Connoisseur of Tits and Apostle of Tit Freedom, personally put those tits back in their imprisoning bra, and then pulled her blouse down and said, "Now carry on with the massage, please!"

Wow! That's like Martin Luther prostrating himself before a statue of the Virgin Mary! That's like the Pope personally handing out free condoms and dildos in Vatican Square! That's like radical feminists fighting for higher pay for underpaid men like me!

So, you see, despite what the French say, things can change, and they don't stay the same.

To continue with the episode of the massage (pardon the long diversion on tits and tit freedom, a subject that gets me very passionate), I asked Inul how many customers she had

had, and she said, none yesterday, and only one today.

She says she hasn't screwed anyone but her pacar or boy friend, and wants to screw me (though she seemed to partly back out when she saw my cock, saying her cunt was too small or kecil). I think I might indeed take up her offer . . . for I am fascinated by her talkative charm, and I want to get to know more of it and her. Indeed, New York in August — the place where I am supposed to go next — bores me compared to this. Everything bores me compared to this.

So this woman, Inul, who could get lost in a dictionary or a kamus or be absorbed in squeezing out one of my blackheads, of her own initiative — I find the kindness and caring in that gesture to be infinitely touching — while I diddled the outer third of her cunt with my middle finger, right in the middle of the massage. Who was so fascinated by English words she would ask me their meanings.

"Apa 'fuck me'?" she once asked. Meaning: "What is the meaning of "fuck me"?" I hadn't used the words with her, for I am generally far more restrained and polite (as they say) in my speech than I am in my writings; in writing, I feel I am entitled to all the freedom the world has to offer its free and fearless writers, whereas in speech, I am shy and "proper". She must have heard the word from somewhere else, and she seemed to have a fascination with learning language, especially the English language and its seamier words.

That evening, I have an Indonesian lesson with Jack the Language Teacher, whose full name, he tells me, is Dear Jack, at which I have to suppress a laugh, for I think him to be no john (it turns out the name is spelled DerJack, which is about the same thing, and how would a person address him affectionately, or begin a letter to him: Dear DerJack? Or Dear Dear Jack?). He's touched by something I say, and I have been having my first real conversation in some days (for a big city can be quite lonely for a shy stranger like me), so I decide to take him out to eat Indian food. It's about 7 pm now, past dusk in Jakarta, neon lights and gas lamps burning brightly as the city is transformed into a night spot, and on a brainwave, I decide to ask the taxi to stop by the massage parlor, pick up Inul, and take her along for dinner.

It is a fine and upscale restaurant, in central Jakarta, on a street where many tourist hotels are; it is a cross between a temple and an art gallery. We order a few dishes like Boneless Chicken Bhuna and Prawn Ginger Masala. Jack enjoys the food immensely, while Inul says nobody in her entire life has taken out to a restaurant as good as this and treated her to food as good as this — a statement that warms my heart, an excellent dinner for three having cost me a mere fifteen dollars, a rare splurge for me in Indonesia and yet so modest compared to New York prices. Afterwards, all of us return to my hotel room, Jack leaves after awhile, and Inul lingers on. Of her own accord, she goes to the bed and lies on it. I kiss her . . . Suddenly, she starts chanting, her eyes spitting fire, "Fuck fuckfuck fuckfuck!"

I burst out laughing. Then I remember that in the massage parlor, she had begged me not to kiss her, because it was making her too horny; had this one minute of kissing so inflamed her as to provoke this outburst of barroom language?

And then, responding to my laughter, her face becomes a pleading one, as she issues a heartrending, single, "Fuck?"

I don't answer, for I would like to postpone this to another time.

However, even after I have refused her, we get distracted once again by the kissing and our passion. Too aroused now, and forgetting my wounded cock, I ask her, "Pulang or fuck?" (meaning, "Do you want to go home now, or do you want to fuck?"); and she answers gleefully, "Fuck!" and within seconds, strips off her clothes and lies on the bed, waiting eagerly for me. And now, I cannot back out; I have to do what a man is expected to do.

It seems I have a fatal (or non-fatal) attraction to women who are attracted to me. Almost as if there is an underlying, deep current of diffidence and skepticism in my system which asks: what kind of woman could *possibly* be interested in me?

When she tells Jack that from my eyes, and from my polite manners, she knows I am a good man, quite unlike her usual massage customers, I am a little skeptical; I don't know whether this statement is obvious flattery with intent to get closer to me and make more profit out of me, or if it is comes straight from her heart. I wish I were more secure about this, but I am not. And I know in that world of supermen and superwomen, of highly realized, enlightened, and advanced human beings, the brave new world of super-beings which many Americans and my ex-wife inhabit and are full-fledged members of, that such a question is completely irrelevant. To them, it is what we think of ourselves that is important, and my anxious concern about what other people, especially women, really think about me is a weak and foolish way to live. (Well, screw them.)

Even as I look at her lying naked on the bed, wondering whether to proceed, the rabbit eyes, so alive and moving and clear and honest and gripping, get me. And also the "fuck me, fuck me, fuck me," uttered rhythmically, as in the hypnotic throes of a hip-swaying, dangdut song. I yield.

I followed this first and unexpected fuck at my hotel with a visit to her massage place the next day. As she massaged me, she confided to me that getting massaged too often wasn't good for you, that one shouldn't do it more than once a week or fortnight. I agreed with her in principle, explaining that I had come today not because I needed a massage, but because I had been feeling a bit depressed this morning and wanted to see her — to be energized by some of her infectious vitality. What she needs to be given a medal for: the difficulty of communication doesn't stop her, she truly keeps on and on, talking and talking, and attempting to explain patiently, word by word, what I don't understand. This little-educated woman has the passion to communicate, and she has heart. How unlike Christ's command the world is. For those who have so little give so much; while those who have so much give so little.

I told her I had to leave Indonesia soon and return to the

U.S. to take my kids on a holiday.

She let out a piteous moan, like the cry of a child (I have to admit a part of me wonders if she is just a good actress who repeats the same story to everyone, but it is not an overpowering thought). And she said, referring to herself in the third person, "But what about Inul? Inul has to be here alone without you?" One of the most touching statements anyone has ever made to me, in my life, and whenever I remember those words, I am filled with a desire to find her again, to search all of Indonesia, trekking through every one of its villages if need be to locate her and find out if she needs me still, and if she does, here I am, at her service, her love slave forever.

Anyway, what really blew me was her reply to my question, on my next visit to her massage parlor, about why her tits were so small.

She said her baby had drunk her milk and in the process shrunk her breasts–her only baby who had died one year back. Without even a request from me, she lifted her blouse, cupped a breast with one hand, squeezed her nipple, and, Presto, a drop of milk came out.

I was surprised and fascinated — spellbound was more like it, for I had never seen anything like this before (being too young when I had access to my mother's breasts to remember anything), never had been given such a gift. So now, I had this sudden yearning to taste her milk, asked her if I could. And she readily said yes, and so I did. It tasted less like cow's milk than like milk reconstituted from nonfat dry milk powder — obviously the design was to discourage overgrown babies like me. But I was very moved by this act of generosity, and also by the fact that her child had died recently, and by the combination of the two.

When I went downstairs on my way out, I passed by a few masseuses who, having no customers, were idly sitting and chatting on the stairs, and tried to confirm from them whether Inul's baby had really died. It's not at all unusual for Indonesians to be pretty glib liars, and a well-executed lie only excites admiration and laughter, almost never social condemnation. So confirming what she had said was somehow important to me. And when they confirmed it, I replied, sadly, "Sorry."

"Why are you sorry?" one of them asked, looking mildly bewildered.

"Because it makes me sad to hear her baby died," I said, puzzled by the question.

"Oh," they laughed. "Because she is your *wife?*"

I was puzzled by their apparent heartlessness. It would have pained me to hear from any woman that her baby had died as recently as a year back. Though admittedly, with Inul, it was more poignant because she had let me be the baby for a minute, had let me, with her endless generosity and love, suck the milk that rightfully belonged to that tragically absent and prematurely dead baby. Yes, for just a few seconds, she had let me be her baby — such a leap from New York State Law on the subject of the proper behavior of masseuses with their customers.

EAST JAVA AND THE PADLOCKING OF WOMEN'S PRIVATE PARTS

When I saw the headlines, I was shocked. How could this be happening in Indonesia, an amazingly tolerant and sweet-natured and sensual country, a country with some of the best and happiest people in the world? For it was a country which, despite being overwhelmingly Muslim, could teach a few other non-Muslim countries the right attitude to life. But the headlines were clear: In Batu, a mountain resort surrounded by volcanoes, and situated south of the coastal city of Surabaya in East Java, a nearly all-Muslim region, a town council dominated by conservative Muslims had passed an order requiring masseuses to work with padlocks around their waists. Yes, you heard it right: the women would, during their working hours, have their womanhood corseted, contained, arrested, and commandeered by the authorities, by Big Brother no less. To be fair, even "conservatives" in Indonesia are exceptionally liberal by Saudi Arabian standards, because the town council didn't try to stop the women from driving, talking to men, going around in public without veils, or even massaging men; the rule was apparently designed *just* to prevent them from having sex with their massage customers. Which is such a reasonable and modest goal, when you compare Indonesia to certain other countries, where a woman could be arrested and be subjected to a public lashing simply for being *seen* with a male who was unrelated to her.

Still, what the news item didn't fully explain was how the padlock could resist the simple expedient of a duplicate key. For if the masseuse really wanted to do it, she could manage to get herself a key, right? And how exactly would she pee? Would she have to get a key each time she needed to go to the toilet?

Anyway, when this story hit the news, the Indonesian Minister for Women's Affairs, herself a woman, condemned the order, saying that this particular method of control was demeaning to women, because it implied that it was *women* who were immoral, instead of being, according to her, the pitiful victims of rampant male lust. She fully agreed that any hanky-panky occurring in massage parlors ought to be stopped, but suggested that the honorable and less demeaning method would be to install closed circuit TV cameras in these establishments.

And I smiled, thinking (with more than a pinch of vanity, as you'll realize from the story that follows): *they are bolting the stable doors after the horses have bolted.*

Let me rewind the narrative a bit, or rather give a flashback to my years of intensive and fanatically frequent massage in New York between 1988 and 2001, when I would undergo at least three massages a week for over ten years from licensed massage therapists without engaging in sex (except for a few truly exceptional times, described in the other book, *The Uncensored Massage: Massage and Sex in America and Elsewhere*). First of all, there would be the big flashing signs in the sky provided by the towel, the blanket, and the mournful, grim demeanor of the masseuse, and the long "Patient Information Form" that she asked you to fill up, as if to prove your character and to provide her with legal remedies should you or a microscopic and sometimes unruly part of you misbehave. And if all that wasn't enough, she just had to say the words "New York State Draping Law," and you knew you would not *want* to have sex with that masseuse in a million years, not even if *she* offered to pay you for it.

But in Asia, especially in Southeast Asia, things are wildly different. Many a bodily issue or phenomenon that Western masseuses regard as logistical problems or legal minefields (a sudden erection, for example, or an emission out of the blue) are simply considered funny by a Southeast Asian masseuse, and excite laughter; and when a Southeast Asian woman laughs, it is as if the warm island sun has risen from the sea or from behind a mountain, the atmosphere loosens up and warms up (and believe me, it is loose enough already). Usually, her companions are within hearing distance in the other cubicles, and when one of them starts laughing, they all start laughing. And even if you are the object of the laughter, you cannot but help smile, unless you are one hell of a prick.

To return to my comment about bolting the stable doors too late (a flippant comment, and I'm being something of an unlicensed standup comic in the rest of this paragraph): I felt that it was really too late for them to introduce padlocked pants, because on four earlier visits to Batu, between 2002 and 2006, I had fucked — or rather, to speak the technical truth — been fucked *by* a few of these masseuses, or at least by those I could get around to, and a handful of them five or six times.

And to think that it all happened thanks to a highly improbable *chain* of accidents, starting with a chance meeting on an airplane returning from Australia with an Indonesian Chinese woman, who had given me her phone number and email address. That in turn had led to a rendezvous in Malang, her home town. At Surabaya airport, arranging a taxi for Malang, a Dutch-planned city situated on a cool plateau between two or three glorious volcanoes, I had decided to share a taxi with a garrulous Malaysian Chinese man, who informed me that once I visited my ladylove, I *ought* to make a side trip to the mountain town of Batu, an hour up from Malang, and a sort of Paradise in the clouds. Which I did after meeting my Chinese friend and making her smile from ear to ear, and in a few other places besides.

Perched at 4,500 feet above sea level, the town of Batu, spreading from a central square and the main mosque and market, actually straddles a valley surrounded by mountains and volcanoes that rise up to 9,000 feet; from one part of the town, when I was there around 2007, you could actually see a smoking volcano that puffed up rocks and smoke every seven minutes or so. Domestic tourists from the plains and from Indonesia's second largest city, Surabaya, drive or bus up for the weekend, but the town has its own year-round residents, schools, and a market in which fresh fruit and vegetables are sold by farmers from the surrounding villages.

Naturally, as the beds in the cheap hotels I slept in were uncomfortable, battered foam beds, and because having to bend over low coffee tables to work on my laptop had hurt my back, I found myself hunting for massage establishments in Batu, and stumbled into them. I knew the difference between a massage establishment and a brothel, of course, and these looked like absolutely genuine massage places — occasionally, a sixtyish middle-class Indonesian couple could be seen leaving these establishments after having received a treatment. So I had no inkling of what was going to happen. Besides, the price was irresistible — on my first visit in 2002, it was 15,000 rupiah for an hour — or $1.50 at the then-prevailing exchange rate, which was terrific even in a country where basic local meals, a fried rice with beef or a mie goreng or fried noodles, for example, could be had for sixty cents or less.

And it did start as a proper massage, with me directing them to the parts of my body where I was hurting the most (back, shoulders, arms). But at some point, what with the proximity and tenderness of the masseuse, my desire revealed itself (it popped up against my wishes, and to my embarrassment) and the masseuse laughed, and petted the misbehaving object, sometimes using the moment of laughter to take a better look at it and make a rather appreciative comment. Which, as tends to happen with us insecure and vain men, had the effect of further inflaming my desire and my erection. And thus began my discovery not only that these masseuses could be fucked, but that they were quietly eager and delighted to be, without having overstepped their bounds into seduction or sluttishness (somehow, the chemistry and the built-up heat in each of us caused it; I don't blame either of us). For it seemed that the culture regarded fucking as a wholesome and healthful activity, much as Americans regarded scouting, hiking, jogging, or camping; when one of them had had a good fuck, they would tell their friends, who would cheer them on and celebrate their good luck.

My first massage in Batu, a Traditional Javanese Massage, was just an amusing variation of the "Traditional Balinese Massage" (you notice that the massage is almost always the same, a blend of Swedish, Shiatsu, and oil massage, but the middle word changes to Javanese, if you are in Java, and so on, depending on the island you are on). *Variation*, you ask? So you have been there, done that: the Alexander Technique, The Philip, Darius, Cyrus, and UpyourAnus Techniques, Rolfing and Golfing, and Lomi-Lomi and Momi-Momi, every variation under the sun. But I bet you haven't had the Noor Up Your Ass Massage, which I have.

And the total price including tips: $5.

Picture this: I am lying face down on the massage table, naked as the day I was born, and my legs spread at a thirty-degree angle because my masseuse, Noor, has ordered me to do so; and when a fully dressed woman orders a naked man to do something, he better obey her orders. My cock is erect and peeping out from between my spread legs, easily visible to her. She has climbed up on the massage table, her knees resting between my legs just below my bottom, and as she bends forward and backward to massage my mid-back, up and down, the tails of her doctor's coat (yes, they dress professionally in this joint, you better not entertain impure thoughts!) sweep up and down the back of my penis, balls, and buttocks, it's almost as if I am being tickled with feathers, sometimes the edge of the coat is driving up my anal divide, and she isn't even conscious of all this, doesn't even know that any second now I am going to have a huge ejaculation, to prevent which I am furiously engaging my brain in mathematics exercises which I haven't attempted since my high school final Mathematics exam: dividing and multiplying large numbers, remembering algebraic formulas, and giving myself all the other mental distractions that might delay ejaculation, including the most effective one: visualizing my former mother-in-law.

The next day, I visit a new establishment: Pijat Tradisional (what a laugh that their *traditional* massage occurs in the nude — in which case, it must be considered a radical terrorist for a customer to insist on wearing clothes). Anyway, in the new place, it is Yuni, who is a bit plump but has lush, long hair. She allows me to open her blouse and fondle her tits, which turn out to be unexpectedly massive, firm yet squeezable, and conical, not round hard balloons like those depressing boob-job tits. Indeed I proceed to suck them, and she draws me closer, while she closes her eyes. But after this pleasant and absorbing diversion, I am hard, and hot, and when you are hard and hot, you must be fucked, and or somehow this excess sexual energy must be drained away, or else you are not going to enjoy your massage. You've gone past the Point of Fuckless Pleasure, which is the point of No Return Without Pain; to retreat, at this point, is going to ruin the rest of your day. That's why making you ejaculate, with deft, soft hands or a sensual mouth, is almost the religious central point of Japanese, Korean, and Chinese massages (there are few cultures in the world who are as practical as the Japanese, the Koreans, and the Chinese, the Chinese leaving a triangular cut, starting in the front just above the pubis and ending in the back just above the bottom line, in every baby's baby-suit, so that the baby's excretions can enter the atmosphere instantly and without obstruction). And that is why Japanese and Chinese masseuses are usually mystified by customers like me who refuse the traditional hand or mouth release, their only explanation being that we must be cheapskates trying to save money.

Luckily, what a truly *traditional* climax Yuni is able to offer for her *traditional* massage, which must have been originally invented to enable kings and princes to perform for their wives and mistresses: a *traditional* fuck!

It wasn't the most comfortable fuck, admittedly, the room only half-shielded by a swinging door that was unlocked, with the masseuse's slippers placed just outside the door to signal that no one was to enter (a signal that was always honored, by the way). And the massage table on which we did the deed was not the most comfortable, being narrow and draped only with a bed sheet. Also, we were in a hurry to finish before our time was up. Still, there is also an added sexual excitement about doing dangerous things, added to which our need was pressing enough that both of us left the room grateful and smiling.

My second victim (or rather, as I see it now, if anyone was the victim, it was I), was big-breasted Sinta (Indonesian for Sita, the wife of the Hindu god Rama). The very warmth with which she received me, the broad smiles and intimacy with which she massaged me, the passion with which she tongue-kissed me — Indonesian women are among the world's greatest kissers, I have rarely met one who was not good at it — I confess to taking the initiative, but as connoisseurs know, and an important French male dignitary in the news reportedly found out to his dismay, it takes two to tango, to tongue-kiss, and to perform 69. Added to which, the alacrity with which she helped me unbutton her clothes, the way she drew my head closer to her breasts when I started to suck them . . . how could I have resisted?

During my next few visits to Indonesia, in the next five years, I made three more trips to Batu, each lasting about twelve days, and during this period, the price of the massage jumped from $1.50 to $2.50 and then to $3.50 per hour (a dizzying rate of inflation percentagewise, yet thankfully still affordable to me). Also, during that time, I probably fucked or was fucked by at least ten different masseuses, on average aged around 26, a total of perhaps 25 times.

Two of these massage establishments were located within walking distance of a barbecued duck restaurant called Bebek Buali. I love the taste of roast or barbecued duck, and the duck (like the fucks) could be had for close to peanuts, or around two dollars a plate. Sometimes I would have duck followed by a fuck, and at other times, I would have a fuck followed by duck, though never ever fucking a duck (I must share this at some point, and now is as good a time as any: massages and fucks often leave me hungry, and massages combined with fucks leave me ravenous). It took me some years to realize that countries in which ducks are a regular part of the cuisine are also easy places to get fucked, though I don't know if there is a scientific connection between ducks and fucks.

Once in a while, I would have barbecued whole fresh fish for about two dollars, or there would be lamb satays and curries at other restaurants or warungs (Warung Bethanya being a favorite), or at one of the two Arab restaurants in town. Most of the time, various combinations of chicken and rice, along with a watermelon or avocado milk shake (delicious fruit shakes are amazingly cheap in Java and Bali), did fine; and above all, after the heat of the Javanese plains, I loved the cool fresh air of the town and the fact that in every direction you looked, a glorious vista of mountains, clouds, greenery, sky and the occasional mosque dome or minaret presented a never-ending feast for the senses and balm for the soul.

And here's the funny thing I discovered at one of these places that had five masseuses. That I began to be passed around. To my increasing disconcertment, the traditional equation in which men passed around a passable lay to their friends had been reversed. As a healthy and recently divorced male, I had sexual needs, no doubt (indeed, there's no aphrodisiac like a recent divorce), but I was also looking for affection. I am a sucker for affection, you see. For love. I roam the world looking for a signal that a woman needs me and wants to have me at any cost. (Sometimes, I do find such women, but unfortunately soon discover, after the initial period of blind passion and amore, that they are not the sort of women I want as long-term partners; it is part of that old cosmic joke of God's to make people desire you who you don't desire in return, and vice versa.)

I may have felt somewhat flattered at first, but soon began to feel mildly uneasy if not threatened that a handful of these Indonesian women, reasonably devout Muslims no doubt (all of the twelve except the single Balinese woman, a Hindu who had been cast out of Balinese society for causing what she described as a *ribut* or a social disturbance), were taking on a traditionally male role in looking at me as if I were a piece of meat and passing me around. And speaking of a male role, and there's why the expression "fucked by" came up earlier in the book — two or three of them pressured me to do it woman-on-top style. My own preference has always been for man-on-top, or side-by-side, or kneeling while the woman is on the edge of the bed, or a rear entry, or some combination of these. But these women, knowing the kind of control and pleasure they can extract from a man (or his dick) in the female superior position, strongly urged, and sometimes succeeded, in persuading me to make an exception for them. Yes, the horses had bolted, and they had ridden me too, in addition to being rid by me.

I don't think I was anything special, except that I was a customer who was willing to be fucked and to fuck them back with tenderness, and possibly, my being a foreigner meant they could hope that no one in the community discovered their secret dalliances.

But to return to the main issue or controversy, and why I think the media coverage of this issue skirts the real, deeper truth: Indonesia is one of those countries where women, once they have had babies and have lost their figures (sometimes, even if they have had babies and have maintained their figures, or if they have put on a bit of weight), are sexually neglected by the virile male population, which is often fixated on young meat, on pussy that is from 17 to 24 years old (and yes, this is true of married men too; Indonesians are justly reputed for their extramarital activities, and they almost never feel guilty about them — it is almost, in the case of men, a condition of their masculinity, and the only precaution to be taken is to be careful not to be caught in the act by their wives). So a 25-year-old woman who is a mother or who has been abandoned or is sexually neglected by her husband or lover can find it difficult to have her sexual needs met. In their thirties when, paradoxically, women's sexual drive reaches its peak (whereas men's sex drive has started to decline from age 19 onwards), it can get even harder for them to feel wanted and to get the physical loving they need.

And believe me, what was happening between me and these women was not prostitution by any definition except by the broad definition according to which all human beings are prostitutes, in that we *use* each other, and obtain some form of *gratification* — whether security, love, sex, money, power, career advancement, friendship, intellectual stimulation, revenge, ideological satisfaction, or appreciation — from *every interpersonal transaction* not required by law or obligation (when we don't, we are disappointed, and will not repeat that transaction with the same individual). Because by any realistic standard, including Indonesian standards, what I tipped them was barely more than the tip for a good massage (my *total* payment, the massage fee and tip included, would have barely made the suggested *tip* on a thirty-dollar restaurant meal in New York). It could not therefore be argued that they were selling sex, for they were merely getting paid fair wages for a good massage, even by Indonesian standards. It was obvious that they were giving away the sex for free, simply because they were enjoying it, and they had needs just like the men.

I began to realize that these women treated each other like real sisters, real sisters who withheld nothing from each other, told each other everything, shared everything. To get a sense of the atmosphere: Once, after a massage, three of them were sitting around relaxing in their lounge-cum-kitchen, one of them munching on a snack of fried bananas, and as I passed by, they asked me to sit down and join them. As the only free seat was next to Yanti, another masseuse I had once used (but not fucked), even as I chatted with them, I was holding hands with and fondling Yanti's breasts. (In Indonesia, to be within intimate reach of a sexually hot woman's breast and not to fondle it seemed a criminal waste.) It was absurd and yet beautiful at the same time that they had such a sisterly attitude, and that such a gesture resulted in no catfights. Lina was encouraging me to get massaged by Yanti a second time, and when it turned out that I said no, I preferred Lina, because she was the most passionate, they all laughed. They were all in a raunchy mood, and Lina popped out a breast right in front of the others, and Yanti confessed to me she did indeed have a lot of pussy hair, and I, taking advantage of the liberal nature of the conversation, asked Cita if she swallowed, to which she replied no, she spat.

I realize in hindsight that this was possible because the women ran the show without male gatekeepers. This is not often the case; in many other places in Indonesia, and particularly in Bali, there are male gatekeepers, who utter the words "security"(meaning some security guard has to be paid off) and "ratus"(meaning 100,000, a multiple of which is supposedly the required fee) with solemn seriousness, as if the words themselves gave them an orgasm, and when the "system" is in place, the women are not truly free beings, and it is a game from which men profit more than the women for doing nothing other than providing the "protection" and ensuring an inflation in the prices. In such a situation, a woman is not free to be her true self.

Back to the situation at Lina's massage joint: after I repeatedly refused Lina's suggestion that I fuck Yanti, because she didn't turn me on, and neither did her massage technique (and no matter what the other qualities of a masseuse, when my body is aching, I insist on a good massage first), this annoyed Lina. Because Lina had "lost face" — this very Asian phenomenon that I, a Westerner, was unaware of. She had lost face with her friend, who was almost like her sister.

After this, I did not feel welcome there anymore. Which saddened me a bit, but anyway, I had been due to leave the country in the next two or three days. It took almost 2.5 years for me to make my next trip to Batu, and now I was partly anxious to investigate the padlock story. Here are my notes, written in the hotel after two meetings with them:

6 p.m. A simultaneous wailing from three mosques, quite a production, but it's a somewhat more mellifluous, less angry and cantankerous one than in some other Third World countries.

It was a long-awaited moment. I had come here to investigate the chastity belts, and was greeted at the door by Lina, who led me into the room after a tongue-kiss while guiding my hand and placing it over her breast — yes, she placing my hand on her breast and holding it there with her hand — a gesture I found to be incredibly affectionate and touching, after all these years. And when I entered the room, she implanted a kiss on my chest and on my trousers just over where my aroused penis lay, waiting to be released from its confines. Feeling excited and moved by her unstinting welcome, I reached under her blouse and fondled her nipples and later, her buttocks.

After a couple more minutes of fooling around, her way of giving me a warm welcome, she decided to place me under the care of a fat and short masseuse, apparently because she was busy with another customer. This puzzled me. When the fat one entered, I was resistant, and told her I would like to have Lina. But I was given a bureaucratic reason for the change, saying her name had already been entered in the register. Reluctantly, I understood: possibly they had introduced some new egalitarian system by which the women were assigned customers as their number came up, thus ensuring that no single masseuse was overly favored?

Another masseuse assured me that I would be allowed to see Lina the next day, and it seemed to be the general agreement that tomorrow I would fuck Lina, because I clearly informed the fat lady that I would not have any ciki-ciki or pompom (local slang for fucking) with her. Later, I would realize that the lie, which is an Asian device for saving face, could also have been a matter of hiding the fact of Lina's having her period.

In the room, the fat masseuse assured me that the system of locks had stopped a month back, and she readily showed me her padlock-less pussy — hairy, it turned out — which I, out of politeness (it would have been real bad form to insult her at this time, having already rejected her request for a fuck, while implying that Lina was my preference), felt, allowing a probing finger enter half a centimeter into her vaginal opening.

Yes, I had landed in East Java on a literary-moral mission for mankind, and felt delighted to report that so far, the sexuality of these women had not been significantly strangled by the bumbling attempts of those misguided males.

The next day, Lina had her turn with me, and we had our reconciliatory fuck, though some of the earlier spark had gone, because we had changed, I perhaps more than she had. (And, reflecting back on what had happened the last time— her attempt to share me with others—I began to realize that she may have partly meant to send me a message: "Don't get emotionally attached to me, it is just a fuck, we are just having a good time." It would have been perfectly in character for her to think like that.)

Returning to the subject of the repression of women's sexual freedom through the use of padlocked pants or any other heavy-handed method, consider this: It is not men's sexual decadence, or even women's, that is at fault: this fault-finding between the two sexes is ridiculous, and must end, because it is a complete diversion from the real issue. The real issue is that in various Third World countries, societies exist, or have been created, in which sexual provocation is increasingly in the air, transmitted by modern communication, music, film, the Internet, travel, the shrinking of international boundaries, geographical as well as cultural, as well as freely available porn VCDs and DVDs (a recent hardcover porn video starring three Indonesian celebrities has been seen by 40 million people, or nearly half the adult population). For all this increased provocation and seeming liberalization, these societies include millions of men as well as women who have no legal or easily available outlets for their natural sexual needs, and must therefore invent covert subterfuges and devices for having these needs met. Until this issue is addressed, every vaginal padlock will merely end up producing its own duplicate key.

Men of the World, wake up and realize this: you will never succeed in the padlocking of desire, whether men's desire or women's. Or, to conclude with an ancient Sumerian poem, which reflects a timeless question that must always figure in policy considerations:

As for me, Inanna,
Who will plow my vulva?
Who will plow my high field?
Who will plow my wet ground?

Yes, indeed. So long as the world is blessed with vulvas, someone or the other will have to plow them. And for a brief while, while I was capable, I was more than happy to shoulder a microscopic fraction of this burden.

BEHIND THE NO HANKY-PANKY DOOR: MASSAGING YOUR BABY IN VIETNAM

Shift the scene to Vietnam, which after four decades is taking baby steps towards rejoining the informal confederation of its neighbors known as Pleasurelandia.

Vietnam is one of the most beautiful countries in the world, blessed by nature, and also by the fertility of its population. It is home to a proud people, being the only country in world history that has achieved a military victory over two of the world's superpowers (or near-superpowers): the United States and China. I have known more Vietnamese outside Vietnam than inside, and nearly all the Vietnamese I have known outside Vietnam have been women, and, at the risk of generalizing (you could not write a book like this about a huge part of the universe without doing a lot of generalizing — I make no claims to being a specialist on any subject), there are four or five qualities or characteristics that I admire in them: the musicality of their language, which is the most sensual of the three tonal languages I know, especially when spoken by its women; the toughness of their constitutions, which partly explains to me why they survived a 15-year war with the world's foremost superpower; their sense of humor and big smiles (a staccato "I. Love.You; You. Love. Money!!!" will make them laugh every time); and their anti-imperialist, anti-capitalist, and utterly endearing hatred of panties, and their tendency to go around wearing pajamas under which they are completely naked.

In Vietnam itself, possibly because of the long era of Communist rule, moral policing, and fear, and despite a mushrooming of massage joints, you can never be sure what exactly you are getting with a Vietnamese massage. Whatever it is, it is often going to be a bit less than promised, because the chief objective is quick money — far more money than the often untrained practitioners would make at another comparable occupation in a week or sometimes, a month.

On my first visit to Saigon, a charming city with French architecture, innumerable cafes and an immense motorcycle-borne population, a couple of hotel massages in the hotels costing around $20 to $25 a night had given me the privilege of being massaged by an exceptionally beautiful young woman, possibly around 22, straddling me while wearing thin white silk shorts. The shorts formed an artistic camel-toe of her cleft, with an artistry that Michelangelo would have been proud of, even though his personal preference was guys. The camel-toe and the shorts left little to the imagination; to add spice to the red-hot chili of her outfit, she also wore an attractive, minimalist white blouse (the white to signal a pseudo-medical professionalism and purity, I presume). It seemed to be the standard uniform in those hotel massage joints (these were one or two-star hotels), and it was about as convincing as Tenth Avenue junkie hookers dressed in Florence Nightingale outfits. Another feature of this and most massage places in Vietnam: the door to your room or booth is a No Hanky PankyDoor with a peephole, or a partially transparent glass door, or a wooden or other screen below or above or through which the massager and massaged can be observed. Probably this conveys the aura of supervision, though nothing prevents the supervisor from being "in" on the game, permitting almost anything, and taking a cut from the proceeds.

The Saigon masseuse straddled my buttocks or my silk-shorts covered penis for 30–40 minutes while she used her hands to excite — I mean to "massage" — other parts of me. Whatever the brochure had claimed it to be, this massage was pure tantalization: exquisite and divine, but tantalization and arousal to the limit. If I were the kind of guy who would ejaculate on the excitement alone — as indeed I was, when I was a sexually starving teenager — I might have ejaculated five times in fifty minutes. But she was also shrewd enough as to cease her erotic pressure just seconds before the point of no return. Again, the goal was to exercise high-quality persuasion so that I would accept an extra: a hand job or a blow job, both of which I refused, not even asking her for her rates.

This seemed to be the Saigon specialty: I visited two other massage joints, and the procedure was exactly the same: gorgeous women, exquisite tantalization, and a feeling that without a happy ending or someone to have sex with at the end of it, you might go stark raving mad.

I had a somewhat different Vietnamese massage experience at a hill resort town north of Saigon called Dalat, four thousand feet above sea level and sometimes called the French Alps of Vietnam for its architecture, rolling green hills and blue mountains in the distance, and its lakes. Here, I decided to visit an old hotel with a "sauna and massage" advertised as being 100,000 dong or seven dollars a massage. I never saw the sauna, and still don't know whether there really is one: I have realized that in Vietnam, signboards are meant to be decorative, and may have no direct connection with reality: a place that advertises fried rice for 20,000 dong on its door might refuse to sell fried rice, or even flied lice, for anything less than 40,000 dong.

Paying the money in advance at the ground-floor reception, I was dispatched up an elevator to meet my would-be Makers: I mean my masseuses.

Given a choice of two masseuses, I chose the older, less sexy masseuse. First, because the sexy and pretty one had long nails — which would inhibit her ability to give me a serious massage without resulting in scratches or cuts to my skin. Second, because an older, less pretty masseuse possibly had more experience and was less likely to believe that the world owed her a living just because she was young and beautiful. And I really needed someone to work on my muscles: pain relief had priority over sexual need.

Once we were in the room, she gave me a decent massage, though in fits and starts, and only when I repeatedly made it clear to her that I would not like my "baby" massaged, but that I had real body pains and needed a real massage. She kept persuading me, offering the baby massage for a mere twenty-five dollars (or five times the cost of the body massage itself), but I refused.

At some point — I now fail to remember what the provocation was, and don't think that I used an old trick and asked her if she had any hair down there — she lowered her short skirt to reveal a massive bush about the size of Chad. What was she trying to do? Seduce me? Get me horny because I wasn't feeling that horny today, being focused entirely on my pain? It was a massive bush, a bush of the kind that staggers Butters, the touchingly delightful kid in the television series *South Park*. Butters, having been shown a sex education clip in school, cannot help but keep muttering, again and again, "That bush! Why that *bush*?!"

And that's what I thought too. I asked, "Why don't you shave it?" She seemed taken aback by my suggestion, and was disappointed that her display of her stupendous bush had not led me to go in for her twenty-five dollar "baby massage." Imagine the irony: she was willing to give a hand job or a blow job to one American dong at the mind-blowing exchange rate of 500,000 Vietnamese dongs (or $25) per American dong. Still, it was a lot cheaper than taking her to a Broadway show (which *South Park* reveals to be a secret technique for getting blow jobs). Also, in showing me her bush, she had shown me a bit of her humanity — which is what you find a lot of in Vietnam: humanity, vulnerability. And which I found a lot less of in China.

For my third massage in Dalat, I decided to try a four-star hotel with a panoramic view of the city, the lake, and the surrounding mountains, one which had a large sauna cum massage establishment in its basement, with a landscaped Japanese garden and a small pool with lotus plants and flowers floating on it. It was more expensive, but I reasoned that a four-star hotel would have better supervision and have well-trained masseuses — who would be restrained from trying extortionate tactics on the customers.

Yes, this was a real sauna, and after changing, in a locker room, into silk shorts provided by the hotel, I walked through a sauna and whirlpool area (where a couple of naked possibly Japanese customers were enjoying themselves) to the massage area, where a lovely possibly 25-year-old woman named Kim greeted me warmly and followed me to the massage cubicle with the regulation No Hanky Panky Peephole.

Kim ordered me to remove my shorts, and I plopped, naked, onto the massage table, facing down.

At which Kim, though she placed a towel over my buttocks, climbed onto the table, lowered the towel, and sat on my buttocks with her short white skirt, brief panties, and silky legs and buttocks, the panties covering so little of her delicious parts that I had the sense that she was riding me bareback, like Lady Godiva, riding my ass.

It was an incredibly erotic sensation, and my penis went from 0 to a theoretical 90 in around ten seconds, and stayed there for a while as she hurried through a back massage and asked me the Great Vietnamese Question, one that no longer made me laugh, but just smile: "Want massage for baby?"

I didn't answer, but made her continue with the back massage, finally explaining that I was a writer and had extra back pains that needed massaging, and that was my priority.

She took it gracefully, and was a good sport about it. She

kept trying her bit to arouse me, however, and allowed me to slide my fingers under her panties, and to feel her soft but prominent orchid, yes, a clitoris that was in bloom, the proud clitty of a woman who was either blooming, or who was strumming her guitar every night without fail, and every spare moment she could get. And when I turned over, she now repeated her question "Massage baby? No?" even as she actually massaged The (Now Erect) Baby. She then made a sign, pointing to my cock, as if to suggest that my cock was as thick as her arm — a piece of bald flattery that nevertheless improved her chances of success with insecure men like me.

Believe it or not: she posed the exact same question to me, in Braille, around ten times. She would do this for a few delicious seconds, say about ten or fifteen seconds, her hand making three up and down movements on my penis, and then stop. And after another short massage interval, she would do it again. How could I refuse such delicious free ministrations from such a gorgeous young Vietnamese woman, one who looked like a model? Do I refuse free tastings of wine or cheese at a supermarket or a wine shop? Never. (I will even eat the crackers and the sample slices of cake, at times.) And what she was offering me was "samples" or "previews" of something far superior to wine and cheese, so I kept pretending to be in a "consideration" mode, as if I might indeed change my mind if the sample happened to be good enough. She was smart enough not to overdo it, or else her question might have been answered by a shower of gratitude, along with my smartass response, "Oh, oh, oh, my God! Oh my Buddha! *No*, thank you, I think I'll pass!" She also lowered her skirt to show me her small pussy, mildly hairy and nothing like the massive thick bush of the masseuse at the earlier joint. Once again, I'm trying to remember why exactly she did this: was it to arouse me, or perhaps I had asked her if she had hair down there? (A great question that works at least one-third to half the time.)

Yes, she gave me ten previews of her "baby" massage, in the form of questions in Braille, all delivered with a smile (oh, what a sport!). I now wish she had also asked me "Want a fuck?" in Braille — ten times. Too delicious to imagine: my penis brushing against that glorious orchid ten times as I pretended to ponder her question and make a considered decision. So delicious, indeed, that I must stop writing this for a few minutes.

[I wonder what some in the West would have thought of her criminal behavior in having violated me well before she had obtained my permission with The Essential 164 questions; even if you assigned a value of three questions to each of the ten questions that she put to me in Braille, it still leaves her 134 questions short.]

And then the massage ended, and she led me out of the massage room to the locker room, holding my hand as if she were my lover. And all for a $2.50 tip! I was really touched by that, and really would have liked to get to know her better; but I knew that, what with my time constraints and life constraints, such a prospect was close to impossible. It was only when I decided to use the sauna and whirlpool that I was able to soften my hardon; still, I went home vaguely horny, thinking that I might have to "baby massage" myself . . . with my own sorry hand (the most politically incorrect act according to my value system) . . . if I was going to get some sleep! Luckily, I was able to sleep with no trouble.

The next morning, all my body pains were still there, and I was still feeling like something the cat dragged in. The sauna and whirlpool had merely dispersed and disguised my pains for a few hours and allowed me to sleep.

Still, the episode had left me with an internal smile.

My fourth massage, back in Saigon, was in an establishment on one of those streets heavily populated by Western tourists, with cheap sidewalk beer joints (50 cents a beer) alternating with budget hotels and massage parlors. Every 30 yards or so you ran into one or two young women, sometimes quite pretty, handing out fliers to passersby and sometimes holding them by the hand to persuade them to come on inside. Having just made a long bus trip over a partly bumpy road, I chose an establishment that had a "discount" massage for 100,000 dong or around six dollars an hour, and only after getting an assurance that I was going to get *only* a massage. Once inside, I was assigned an older, serious, un-pretty masseuse in her late twenties (most of the others were pretty and in their early twenties). She turned out to be new, afraid, and rather amazed that I could speak a few words of Vietnamese (by then), and was asking for specific body parts to be massaged. However, as she knew not a word of English, I was assigned a substitute, a younger, prettier girl who seemed compassionate, indescribably sweet and had that kind of living, breathing, warm satin skin that I have only found amongst a certain kind of Vietnamese woman — I have no idea what their recipe for creating such skin is, but it can be incredibly comforting just to touch it. (Later, she told me she was from the Mekong Delta.)

She was wearing medium-short shorts, light but not too thin, and she started by straddling my towel-covered buttocks, unconcerned that the towel was beginning to slip away — another infinitely comforting sign that this massage was going to be intimate and not too prudish.

And as she did so, some of her thigh skin touched my buttocks and lower back. And then she did something even more arousing. I had pointed to the area on my back that is just above and to the side of my armpits — they are among my most sore spots, and they sometimes need fifteen minutes of massage for me to even begin to feel better. She took my hands and placed them on the soft skin of her *inner* thighs. As if by this method, she had better access to massage my shoulder joints and the back muscles adjacent to them. Which indeed she had; but what about *my* access, my fingers occasionally touching her shorts and skin that was just two inches from her womanly center?

So my manhood was aroused, and as she continued with the massage, she had a nice view of my aroused state, and no doubt planned her next strategic move.

It was to ask me to turn over and then to ask to massage

my head and face. I said: Why not my legs first? She replied: Okay, I will do that, but first I need to do the head and the face. She continued doing this forever, sometimes bending her face for me to kiss it: that was how aroused, affectionate, and grateful I was feeling. She would only let me kiss her face, not her lips — and I accepted her terms. I had also begun to play with her hair, and I was enjoying this: her hair wasn't thick, but silky, and I also derive an indescribable erotic pleasure from running my fingers through a woman's long silky hair.

Here I was, floating in some lower heaven, when, suddenly, she informed me the massage was over.

And I said, "But you haven't massaged my legs!" In other words, if I stopped, I would be left with an incompletely massaged body; and that can feel weird, unbalanced, and could even be dangerous.

She said, "So you want another 60 minutes? Then that will be 280,000 dong." She pointed out the price of a 2-hour massage in the un-discounted menu. In other words, by asking for the two hours, I would shift the entire massage into the undiscounted territory of a two-hour massage, and that was my only choice, as they didn't offer a 90-minute massage on their menu.

Then I realized the second woman had made a sucker out of me. And it hadn't been the first time this had happened.

So be it. It was a one-of-a-kind experience. And if you're in Vietnam, remember that What You See on the Menu is not necessarily What You Get. If you are sure you need a massage and just a massage, take a plane to Thailand or a bus to Phnom Penh, Cambodia.

WACKY ASIAN MASSAGES IN CHINA AND ELSEWHERE

China is a huge country, and a diverse country that was in the news recently for its Communist party officials who had been participating in sex orgies; when you repress the sexuality of so large a country, and of so natural and practical a people, you can expect such a thing to happen. It is reported that there are clubs for swingers, and gigolo services for wealthy women in the major cities. Though I saw little of any of this during my relatively short stay, I did manage to get a tiny slice of Chinese sexual liberation thanks to having learned to speak around fifty words of Chinese (and a bit more than "Woh thin boo tong" or "I don't understand") by around the fifteenth day of my stay in China.

The Chinese Oh-You Massage

My first massage during my first and only visit to China was in Kunming, a city of broad boulevards at an altitude of 5,000 feet in the tea-growing region of southwestern China. In China, the food is so fresh, so authentic, so varied in its flavors, so reasonably priced — dumplings, Peking duck, seafood hot pot with noodles, pregnant fish — it makes all your senses come alive, but sooner rather than later, you will need a massage, for the mattresses in most budget and mid-level hotels tend to be very thin and somewhat hard. And, walking into a spa-cum-massage joint, an independent wooden building next to my hotel, I was given a locker key by the male receptionist and commanded by the male locker attendant (who looked like a People's Army veteran minus the uniform and the bayonet) to strip and change into a laughably brief pair of shorts. He then directed me to proceed to the steam and massage section, where the women, dressed like nurses in white uniforms, lay in wait to ambush me.

I had paid for the *basic* massage: around fifty yuan, or seven dollars. And, glad to be relieved of my tight shorts, I lay naked under a towel as the masseuse began to massage me.

She didn't speak a word of English, or so I believed, and I not a word of useful Chinese, so we resigned ourselves to our respective roles in the massage, I deciding to take it as it came.

But around fifteen minutes into the massage, the woman, possibly thirty and passably pretty and nice-figured, began exclaiming, "Oh you! Good!" every thirty seconds.

"Oh you! Good!" she kept saying, as I looked at her, mystified, thinking perhaps that the sight of my virile body was giving her an orgasm every thirty seconds (ah, my silly male ego!), and that while the "Oh you!" was an orgasmic exclamation, the 'Good!' was a comment on the quality of the orgasm.

Only after thirty minutes of this did I finally figure out that "Oh-you" was her Chinese pronunciation of "oil" — which, with its two syllables, was too difficult for some Chinese to pronounce. All along, she had been urging me to change my massage to an *oil* massage, which she was better at, and for which her earnings and tips were higher. And also because the "Oh you!" massage was much likelier to culminate in a happy ending for my Little Emperor.

I soon learned that if there is a lesson here in China, it is that illegal pleasure is going to have severe consequences . . . at least on your wallet. A Chinese massage ("health massage") costs from 30 to 50yuan. But an oil massage is anything from 100 to 200 yuan. It's not the extra cost of the oil, but the promise of illicit titillation, of your skin being touched, perhaps sensuously, by a masseuse. Though things are changing, the official line still frowns on sensual pleasure. Wealth, yes; pleasure, no.

In between the austere "Chinese health massage" and the decadent "oil massage", there are a few other offerings in which you are permitted to discard one item of clothing, and the price rises for each item of clothing you are permitted to take off. If you *wish* to take off your clothes, that is.

The problem with this system is that the constant pressure on you to go for more, more, and more disturbs and spoils your pleasure and relaxation, which is the reason you have come to get a massage in the first place. It is like being assaulted nonstop by an insurance salesman while listening to a concert of the Berlin Philharmonic Orchestra.

In modern, far more cosmopolitan and fashionable Shanghai, in a quiet middle-class neighborhood perhaps five miles away from the city centre with its futuristic skyscrapers, I received a reasonably competent massage from a 30-year-old call-in masseuse who confessed to me that she was looking for a white man to give her a baby ("because the baby will be more intelligent"). I was both amused and amazed at the amoral practicality of this statement; she might as well have been looking for a prize bull to mate with her cow.

Thanks to my excursions by tram into middle-class neighborhoods that were not on the tourist trail, I discovered an ordinary-looking massage parlor, a small business, a house with around four rooms and six masseuses of different ages from 22 to 45. Once I entered my assigned room, the laughing 22-year-old masseuse with gorgeous black hair jumped with great alacrity at the opportunity to substitute her initial offer of a happy ending with an all-out fuck, and seemed pretty grateful at the end of it. And so was I, because by then, I had been sex-starved for two weeks, and had come a long way from my days of sanctimonious hypocrisy in New York, when I would have protested that I was a noble being who really would prefer to make love to my wife. It turned out to be a gorgeous, passionate, though not too-long fuck, and she invited me for a return visit; I obliged, the next day. Two fucks in two weeks in a country of 1.3 billion people: a mere droplet in a vast ocean, but it humanized my visit, and was mine and the masseuse's tiny contribution towards the cause of international understanding, peace, and brotherhood. It also made up for my mildly frustrating massages in Kunming.

Hole in the Door Massage

A friend of mine, who is more of an aficionado of sex than of massage, told me he once visited a Phnom Penh massage joint which offered a choice from between a hundred masseuses, many of these young and pretty. And these were the kinds of masseuses who looked more like they liked to work with their pussies than with their hands. So he chose a pretty young masseuse, and the pair headed off to a room with only one thing in his mind: a fuck. In such places, you enter a room, close the door, and during the rest of the massage, the masseuse tries her best with her "massage" to arouse you so you will beg for a fuck, at *her* price, or at close to her price.

Well, he needed no persuasion, and also happens to be quite wealthy, though cheap when he can get away with it; they quickly agreed on a price for the fuck. He had stripped and was on the bed when he noticed a large, round glass-covered hole in the door; in other words, a glass window through which the people walking by, whether the other girls, supervisors, or customers, could see what was going on inside the room.

This upset him until she suggested they turn off the lights and do it; he agreed, believing he'd gotten off rather well.

But I challenged his assessment. After all, much of a man's pleasure from a sexual encounter is visual, and he had been denied that. Second, what if someone decided to focus a flashlight through the hole, or a flashlight and a flash camera, and clicked? The next day, the photograph of his prize American ass would have been all over the front pages of the world's newspapers.

Obviously, this place was a victim of schizophrenic hypocrisy; the hypocritical half had installed the hole in the door so that no hanky-panky could go on, or that they could persuade officials that this was a no-hanky-panky joint; while the pragmatic, greedy, lusty other half had decided to sell sex. Were I to find myself in a room like that, I would walk out right away (unless there were absolutely no other choices for ten miles around), because I cannot even handle a normal, no-hanky-panky massage without the assurance of privacy: I need to be sure that what is going on in the massage room is strictly between me and the masseuse, and no one else's business.

Catfighting Masseuses

In Asia, you might sometimes have to deal with territorial conflicts: when one masseuse decides you are "hers," and all others accept — at which point, changing masseuses can result in high drama. So be warned of the risks — and then, choose to enjoy the proceedings, if that's your preference.

In a certain massage establishment in the Beautiful Country with No Name, I once had to choose between two catfighting masseuses, and it seemed that the object of their catfight was I. It happened thus. Early in my visits to this place, I discovered an absolutely fantastic masseuse, Anna, who was so far superior to the local average that I asked for her on my subsequent visits.

In time, the other masseuses considered me to be hers and hers only. She did not allow me to play with her hair or touch her; nor did she kiss me at my request — the kind of thing that I am impelled to ask for when I start feeling affectionate towards a masseuse. I accepted her refusals with grace, because even without any of these extras, her massage was sublime, a gift, a huge bargain when compared to its price.

For six months, I belonged entirely to Anna. Then, when Anna went to her home town on leave, I was forced to try Belinda, who I discovered to be equally good, and a bit more playful besides, allowing me to play with her glorious long hair, among other things. I now became addicted to Belinda, and when Anna returned from her home town, Belinda rubbed it into her that she had won me, and that I was now hers.

Thereafter, every time Anna looked at me, I could see in her eyes the hurt and anger of betrayal.

For an entire year thereafter, I was assigned exclusively to Belinda. However, showing up once when Belinda was busy, and being desperately in need of a massage, I asked for Anna. Anna not only gave me a fantastic massage, but while she was massaging my head, she rubbed her pussy against my head, pretending that it was accidental. Well, she did indeed have her back against the wall, but neither of us was fooled, for she was doing this repeatedly. So, even as she continued massaging me, I, aroused, reached inside the elastic waistband of her stretch pants and inserted my fingers into her pussy and diddled it. She carried on massaging me silently for nearly seven minutes, in the same position, while I continued diddling her, still pretending that nothing had happened, while I could feel her dripping wet.

This was very exciting to me, and when I turned over, my face up, she also allowed me to play with her hair.

However, on my next visit, it was still assumed that I was Belinda's, and that my one massage with Anna had been an exception on account of Belinda being otherwise occupied. So I returned to Belinda. Anna's anger with me at this "second betrayal" was so unforgiving that she refused to ever massage me again. And I knew that Belinda, who had now begun to massage me even more sexily and to permit me liberties that were previously refused, was doing this partly because of her ongoing catfight with Anna.

Hippo Massage

Indonesia is a huge, multicultural and multi-religious country, so do not expect my general observations about Indonesian massage to apply beyond the islands of Bali and Java, which together contain over half the population. Because the variations in attitudes and prejudices, from across Sumatra in the Northwest to Papua in the extreme east, are huge, and I have no experience whatsoever of massage other than in Java and Bali — except for one brief interlude in Northern

Sumatra's Batak country, on the sparsely populated island of Samosir.

Floating in the middle of one of the largest volcanic lakes in the world, this island is indeed a paradise, except in the matter of massages. For here, where the natives have been completely Christianized, the sexual easiness and relaxed nature of the Javanese and Balinese are not so easily to be found.

Noticing hardly any massage places during my walks around the island, I asked the guest house to call in a masseuse to relieve a really bad back. The woman who showed up was around 50 and was built like a hippopotamus, and the result was only what I could describe as the Hippo Massage, in which my entire body and skeletal structure were rearranged, and every plea to her to reduce her pressure brought forth nothing from her but laughter, and just a thirty-second period of reprieve before she returned to her normal bone-crushing self. Because of her rather forceful and dictatorial manner, it took me some time to realize her hands were rough, the nails uncut and filled with dirt. This meant a risk of skin infection. So at this point, I rebelled and stood firm: I told her she would have to clip her nails and wash her hands with soap, and then return to the massage. Then, I proceeded to lend her my nail clipper. She yielded to my insistence, and was a little less rough for the remainder of the massage.

THE HANDSHAKE: OR, THE MILKING
OF THE INDIAN MALE

Despite appearances, you will discover that India, or at least the world of Indian massage parlors, the ones that have been mushrooming recently in cities like Bangalore, is a very friendly and even Westernized place, because instead of the traditional Indian *namaste* or folded hands greeting, they will offer, on their unofficial menu, a handshake.

Yes, you heard right: a *handshake*. Those of you who think, "Well, what's so unusual or bizarre about a handshake, and why mention it on a menu — let alone on an *unofficial* menu? What's going on here? Why is this bozo making such a big deal of this?" — let me explain with an imaginary but not improbable dialogue, partly in Indian English (which I had an ear for, and which you could not miss if you made many visits to India, as I did, on work).

At this Bangalore massage joint called Satisfaction Spa, disguised as a beauty parlor (there are a few barber's chairs in the deceptive and mainly for show entrance hall, but not the forest of hair on the floor and the vaguely cloying smell of cheap talcum powder that you find in the average Indian barbershop), I enter a little massage cubicle in the rear section of the establishment, following a dusky South Indian girl in a sari and coconut-oiled long hair, some jasmine flowers pinned to a single braid. Her laughing, wily eyes are peering at me with curiosity. (She's possibly around 23, but to describe her as a woman would probably insult her — she's so slim and girl-like)

"Do you want a handshake?" the girl asks, once I am as comfortable as I can be on a somewhat precarious and narrow massage table, one of its legs a bit shorter than the other three.

"Why should I be unfriendly? Of course, yes! I've no objection to shaking your hands," I reply.

"I mean, a shake with *my* hands?" Her face seems nervous, while her smile broadens.

"A milk shake that you'll make with your hands?" I ask, looking flustered.

"*Your* milk, sir."More serious, almost demure.

"Excuse me, but you must have gotten my sex wrong. The last I checked, and that was just a few minutes back, I was a man. So sorry, but I don't think you can rely on me for milk production. Anyway, what do you have against cows? This is India, for godsake! Cows are India's national symbol, and they are all over the place; some of them even volunteer their time to work as traffic cops."

"No, Sir, I shake your *little* hand. The little, itty-bitty hand between your legs. With my big hand."

"Oh, you mean my *short* hand! The natives do indeed have quaint customs, I must say. But why, my dear, could you possibly want to shake that slippery little hand of mine?"

"For the milk, Sir. I mean, for the milk from your pen-neese."

"Milk from my pen-neese? Either you are shockingly innocent, or udderly misinformed. The stuff that spurts out of the full-mast pen-neese, as you call it, is not milk, you know. The milk of human kindness, perhaps, or so I have foolishly yet triumphantly declared in umpteen books. But not milk that is fit for consumption by persons under the age of eighteen."

"I mean, the water from your organ, Sir."

"I don't own an organ, Madam, even though I once owned a mouth organ, and am fond of organ music and of organic food, when it doesn't taste like sawdust; but *if* I did own an organ, I wouldn't place too much reliance on it either for water or for milk."

"I mean your *male* organ, Sir."

"As opposed to my female organ? Anyway, my male organ. Oh, I get it. So you're going to shake it for milk or water?"

"Yes, Sir. With my hand. That's the handshake. That will be 400 rupees extra."

"What?! Get outta here! I have never heard of anyone charging for a handshake! It sounds rather unfriendly, what?!"

"No, Sir, *you* get outta here. Our policy is: No Milk, No Honey."

End of imaginary dialogue, which is a composite from many different snatches of real dialogue, and of actions and policies that are unspoken. Though it makes me wonder: why do these people have to torture themselves with such strained euphemisms for penis when the Indian vocabulary contains a majestic equivalent: lingam? [A short break now for a commercial from our sponsors: Milkmaid Condensed Milk.]

Perhaps this dialogue, from the point of view of the poor girl (she's imaginary, so don't let your heart bleed for her, even though mine does, all the time, having allowed her, even in this *imaginary* dialogue, to utter the stinging last words), is a demonstration of mere technical quibbling, mere spoilt-child banter, the superciliousness of a cosmopolitan foreign visitor towards those Indians from more repressed backgrounds who work in these parlors, and even more so towards the poor lambs who come as customers to these massage parlors, who look so desperate (and when I have been in India longer than two or three weeks, there is no lamb in the world who looks as meek and desperate as I do), so desperate that their sad faces betray their admission that they have no option but to subject themselves to any degrading humiliation the girls have to offer, so long as it is some form of recognition that they are human, with organs, with organs that have needs, with male organs that have special needs, one of which consists of being milked or hand-shaken at least once in a month, if not twice a week weakly (forget the daily milking, that is only for the far luckier cows of India, whose sacred right of teat-illation is enshrined in the Sacred Indian Constitution).

Most Indian massage customers, being too desperate, meekly consent when the girls grimly order them to wear shorts, or to keep their underwear on. What's worse (and this happened to me once at an Ayurvedic joint of the strictly non-milking breed), they are sometimes commanded to wear funny little, tightly tied elongated loincloths or Fat Boy G-Strings, Vedic Xtra-Large G-Strings Pour Homme, sometimes by stern male masseurs (who have been trained to affect the stern expressions of headmasters or headmistresses scolding dirty little boys), and sometimes by masseuses. Who knows how many smelly behinds these loincloths have previously dug deeply into in the process, absorbing into their molecular or atomic innards their noxious body effluents? But the Indian sheep meekly obey, indeed they allow themselves to be subjected to this humiliation, this charade, this infantilization, this shrinking of their manhood or humanity, because they desperately yearn to be touched by a woman or a man (yes, even a man will do sometimes), and also to be milked, if they are lucky enough to be in the right place with a willing milkmaid.

However, at a Bangalore massage joint, with a Manipuri masseuse who had massaged me before, and where they had suddenly and unilaterally introduced these paper G-strings — apparently in response to a recent police instruction, threat, or raid — I argued with the masseuse. I told her it was a childish requirement, reducing me to the status of a small boy, it was like having a shower with a raincoat on, and that I didn't like the fake puritanical gesture in this obviously puritan-defying establishment; I concluded by saying I wasn't going to wear that pansy little male panty even if she paid me to do it. And I won my case, for she was a Manipuri, from a Northeast Indian tribal culture that is much more comfortable with the body, that has significantly more affinity with Thai and Vietnamese culture than with Indian culture. Besides which, she had seen everything that could possibly be seen (not so difficult, because the human species comes in basically two models, with only minor variations of size and elasticity), and it was all natural — as natural as shaking hands, or in this case, shaking *little* hands, which she did with a song in her heart if not on her lips. This is one of the great virtues of the girls who come from the Northeastern hill regions of India, as indeed of most of neighboring Southeast Asia. They are not surprised or threatened — let alone shocked or traumatized — by the human anatomy and have a relaxed, cheerful, and realistic attitude towards life. And they must have laughed at the hypocrisy of ordering their shrunken male customers to wear silly-looking, ill-fitting paper shorts, only to slip them down later in the course of the massage to execute their professional, Wholesome, and Wholly Holy Therapeutic Handshake.

While 98 percent of India is choked by the loin cloth of repression, such micro-sartorial oppression is not the fate of the privileged few who frequent the world of the high class massage parlors and the five-star masseuses of India. Such masseuses flourish in five star hotels and certain exclusive spas with hedonistic auras that have sprung up in Bangalore, other metropolises, and the playgrounds of the super-rich. These masseuses are often imported from Thailand, northeastern India, or countries or states where sex is not a huge taboo, and in fact is considered a healthy and even sacred expression of one's humanity, like a three-martini lunch, a languorous hot bath, a visit to the temple, or a postprandial walk. In these enclaves of privilege, the customers pay sixty to ninety dollars for an hour, or exactly the same as they would pay in New York (but five times as much if you factor in India's far lower cost of living); in return, they are permitted to lie in their glorious nudity under luxurious Turkish towels, towels which are manipulated by the masseuse, and sometimes, according to my upscale Indian informant, the son of a senior police officer, simply lifted away for a bit of necessary and compassionate oxygenation of the pitifully suffocated areas, whereupon a smidgeon of exhibitionism on the part of the customer does not immediately evoke a stern rebuke or a tightening of the screw . . . I mean, of the langoti or Male G-string or such other anti-penile weapon, which may also double as a Weapon of Arse Destruction, Division, or Obstruction. Indeed, there is no langoti or male G-string permitted within a mile of these joints, which follow a strict "Leave Your Neanderthal G-String at the Door" policy. It is all spotless Turkish towels and clean white bed sheets. Why this disparity, this apparent discrimination? Because the customers hail from the Master Class (All Heil!), being the sort of worthies and Eminences who holiday in London and Greece and the Riviera if not *being* from there, or are wealthy and pampered foreign tourists like senior Japanese executives or the author and Indophile Paul Theroux, who could probably pay as much as Governor Eliot Spitzer did for a night with his high class *fillies de joie* and not think twice about it. So it is assumed they've seen it all, and at this steep price will not tolerate being talked down to and in the process to have their "little brothers" shrunk in size and status.

Scene: New Delhi: Having arrived in New Delhi on a cold, windy, and gray February day, after an initial visit to Goa and parts of South India, my body is wracked with pain, for I haven't had a good massage in India for two weeks now, only two of those maddening up-and-down piston-style Ayurvedic massages, rendered mechanically by morose male automatons, a one-style-fits all massage. So I call up the New Delhi Hyatt Hotel, which has masseuses. However, it turns out that like Bombay's Taj Mahal Hotel, they will only massage a *resident* guest (their massage therapists have probably been molested, if not worse, by louts who came in from outside? I wonder).

Thus I find myself racing in a freezing autorickshaw to a middle-class New Delhi colony or neighborhood called Lajpatnagar, to some joint the autorickshaw driver apparently knows, only to be driven round and round in that infernal three-wheeler and to discover that the place has closed. After which, returning to my hotel in disgust and defeat, I call up one of the "home service" advertisements from the *Hindustan Times* classified columns, possibly under the heading of beauty services or "health massage," resigned to being violated or manhandled by a prick — I mean, by a male animal.

"What service do *you* want?" the telephone responds. It is a guy named Bob or Ron, impersonating a loaded, ambiguous voice.

"Massage, and nothing else," I reply, earnestly and emphatically.

The guy who arrives at my hotel, and who from his diminutive height and appearance looks like he might be from the Northern hill regions (Bob or Ron, my foot!), is wearing long hair, dark glasses, and a black leather baseball cap, and jeans so tight it probably takes him about five minutes of rough persuasion to make them to wriggle up his thighs.

He goes to the bathroom to wash, and then, to my astonishment, emerges with his pants off and only in his shirt and v-shaped briefs (the tacky cap and glasses have also luckily disappeared). In consternation, I demand that he puts his pants back on pronto, which he does reluctantly, after explaining that they are tight (yes, poor chap, what a hindrance to blood circulation and to a good massage clothes are, and would I have objected to a masseuse taking off her clothes just to get more comfortable? Me, the bloody sexist?! No, I would have popped a bottle of virtual champagne. How unjust life is!). Sure, his pants are tighter than an ant's vagina, which is why, even with them back on his person, they are at present partly unbuttoned.

Still uncomfortable, I think: I have called him anyway, and I need a massage so badly my muscles are on strike; besides, I will have to pay up regardless. So I lie down and hope for the best. He starts the massage. He's pretty strong, and he knows some good massage strokes. But he's racing through the massage like a doggie after a flung doggie toy, spending about five minutes on each major body part like the back, and the back of the legs. Then I discover his massage is designed to be only half an hour long, which is half of my minimum requirement at this point. So I offer to pay a little extra in return for more time. I keep the towel on to discourage any straying of his hands, and find to my relief that he's gotten the message.

What a joke this incident makes of the usual moralistic and stern response that you often encounter in India, when you ask for a female masseuse, and they look at you with amazement, as if you had just asked them to arrange an orgy involving sheep, transsexuals, and camels. For by frowning on any possibility of closeness between the opposite sexes, by the enforcement of segregation of the sexes, the Indian authorities are in fact not just winking at, but encouraging the flowering of a frustrated or resigned homosexuality among those who are naturally heterosexual — and paradoxically so in a country where homosexuality is absurdly, and anachronistically, a crime that could earn you years of prison time (the law that sent Oscar Wilde to jail still remains on the books in India). Call me prejudiced, but I think you're far better off facilitating healthy heterosexual sex, even to the comically paternalistic degree that Singapore does, rather than forcing purely heterosexual but frustrated men to experiment with homosexual sex — which will only end up making them feel guilty, confused, and perhaps worse.

But how can you explain to someone who doesn't understand your language (while you, bad boy, don't understand his!) that what you're interested in is a pure therapeutic massage, and nothing of a homoerotic or even erotic nature, that in fact you are close to homophobic (if apologetically so) and are only with extreme reluctance allowing another man to touch you because, while male masseurs, mostly untrained, or badly trained, are easily available, getting a woman to massage you in Delhi, or for that matter nearly any part of India except perhaps in the shady beauty parlors of Bombay, is as difficult as getting a date with Cindy Crawford? Especially when the very presence of the man, his outlandish appearance (a leather-and-bondage motorcycle chic hick?) and his corny attempts to seduce you by leaving his pants open ("they're tight," he explains) and almost falling off his hips (and his thought that this is somehow attractive to you) makes your face go red with embarrassment, yet you think of this as a bit of penance or mortification that you must suffer in silence, not for past karmic sins, but for the pain relief your sore muscles so desperately need?

Besides, I couldn't tell him to get out simply because he was a homosexual, could I? That was his personal space and choice, besides which he had no control over his biology and his genetic predisposition, and so long as he did his job with me and nothing more, I could not afford to be guilty of anti-gay prejudice, which is a cruel thing, right?

It was only later I realized that all my lofty idealism was bullshit in this sexually confused and morally messed up country, that I would now have to contend with the smirks of the bellboys, and the distancing of the reception manager, for whom all such idealistic argumentation would be too abstruse and foreign. In their view, the chap who had visited me was a fag, and a fag who flaunted it, and if he was in my room for an hour, and if I hadn't thrown him out — or even more propah, called the cops on him — I was a fag too. Oops, oops, oops!

Also, a darker thought. In India, where any sex outside marriage is closely linked with crime and blackmail, and homosexuality is a crime potentially attracting decades of jail time (unlike pocketing a hundred million dollars in kickbacks, which not only escapes punishment, but on the contrary, in famously spiritual and ultra-moral India, earns you the admiration and envy of fellow Indians), perhaps men like him, having already been abused and subjected to the worst elements of human nature in the trade they practiced, saw in persons like me (yes, despite my being a foreign visitor, I was subject to the laws of the land) a potential victim of blackmail?

Which is why I feel Indians should start training low-paid or unemployed women in the art of massage, thus empowering women and increasing employment, tourism, national health and wellbeing, and the per capita income. And world peace.

Because people who receive massages regularly, from women who are at peace with the human body and compassionate and empathetic towards their customers: they are unlikely to be angry, vicious, unkind, and warlike. Let the Koch brothers and other supercapitalists, instead of spreading hatred and war, work to spread the message of massage in Third World countries and even in the so-called (and sometimes warlike) First World countries. We all could do with a little more compassion, tolerance, and benevolence in our natures

APPENDIX I: A RANDOM CONSUMER GUIDE FOR MEN

By now, you are aware of my prejudices, and these prejudices would naturally influence my subjective comments and recommendations below.

Countries

First, I will speak briefly about massage in various countries, while trying to avoid repeating what has been said elsewhere in this book.

BRITISH MASSAGE: Can be professionally excellent as well as un-Puritanical, especially because, in revolt against one hundred years of Victorian morality — which on historical examination has turned out to be mostly high class hypocrisy — Britons have become looser and more relaxed about sex and the body, and far more so than the average American moralizing masseuse (and if you have any doubt, compare a few British episodes of the television series *The Office* with a few episodes of its American counterpart). The English have come a long way from their oh-so-proper past, and English masseuses, surprisingly, can be sensual, intelligent, technically superb, besides having sense of humor that puts you at ease. Or maybe I was just lucky in the choice of masseuses I found (perhaps around 40-50 massages in all from around 10-14 masseuses). Surely the sensual culture of continental Europe, and the relaxed attitudes of immigrants from Eastern Europe, have also helped to make British massage a sexier and more satisfying affair. I have had technically excellent and gently sensual massages at the St. James Health Club fairly close to Piccadilly.

PHILIPPINES MASSAGE: The residents of the Philippines are a remarkably sensual people in general, despite the influence of Catholicism (I have heard comparisons being made to Filipino women and Indonesian women). The massages that I have received are technically proficient and excellent, but I am also aware of the availability, in places like Cebu and Manila, of lingam massage, which is a specialty, derived from the Indian practice of tantra, and may be described as the Pope or the Emperor of Happy Endings.

CZECH & RUSSIAN MASSAGE: In 1996, I spent six weeks in Prague, and a few days in Karlovy Vary, and I had a few excellent and unintentionally erotic massages in Prague. Unless the masseuse seems to have a professional qualification, which is mentioned on the signboard — in which case the masseuse is likely to be technically proficient and uninhibited, but very much like a nurse — you may end up at a place where sex and blowjobs are part of the menu: and I really mean on a printed menu.

Russian massage can also be technically excellent; for it was probably attached to sports, gymnastics, and athletics, and the Russians' desire, in the Communist era, to win a huge number of Olympic gold medals.

THAILAND: Massage is omnipresent in Thailand, sometimes with four massage joints on just one street block, and an oil massage costs from $10 to $15: and lower in non-tourist areas. I often find the best masseuses in the joints that serve Korean tourists (look for a Korean sign on the signboard) or Japanese customers, or those that give oil massages to Thai customers. Most establishments have a system of giving every masseuse a turn, and a new walk-in customer is usually assigned to the next masseuse on the waiting list, unless *she* wishes to pass, or the customer asks for a specific masseuse. If you are particular, say you have not made up your mind, that you need a moment to catch your breath. During that time, you can make eye contact with a few of the masseuses and *choose* a masseuse who seems warm towards you, and looks energetic, eager, and capable.

CAMBODIAN MASSAGE: Cambodians are sensual Southeast Asians partly restrained by their puritanical and hypocritical culture, so what they do in public and what they do in private are two completely different things. The most important consideration from a Cambodian woman's point of view is this: can someone see us doing what we are doing? If she feels assured of privacy, she would like to have fun, and can be generous indeed.

As for the massage scene, it is possibly the most variable country in the world. You may find some of the most untrained women from the countryside massaging you, and a few of them may be quite good-looking too; I find sometimes that customers choose a masseuse for her looks rather than for the massage itself. From the women's point of view: it's only another job for them, easier and better-paying than being cooks or factory workers. At other times, you may find excellent massages, including oil massages for between $5 and $8 per hour, given by masseuses who have been trained by Thai or foreign teachers. I am reasonably certain the quality jumps when the price jumps by two or three times, but I am not in that price bracket at the moment, so I avoid massages that are expensive by local standards. If you can afford them, try them by all means; but also try their cheapest massages to get a sense of the atmosphere, and whether they seem to be repressed and overly patronizing. Once you figure that out, you might decide to try their more expensive offerings. But once again, in the privacy of a cabin or room, a woman may let loose her Inner

Lucretia Borgia; you'll be surprised how much is possible if you just ask!

Usually, you may have to walk around Phnom Penh, and especially into the side streets, and outside the main tourist areas, and at least a kilometer away from the riverside, to find quality massages at prices between five and eight dollars an hour. Still, untrained or trained, they often bring such softness, laughter, tenderness, and even love to their work that it compensates for the occasional lack of training and makes the massage worth it, especially when you're paying so little. One of the nicest gestures a Cambodian or Indonesian masseuse can make towards me is to rest a hand on a part of my body, or to hold my hand tenderly with her free hand while she is using the other hand to massage a different part of the body. That apparently inert hand is passing on love energy to me: and I am hungry for every bit of it.

VIETNAMESE MASSAGE: A world of excitement, of variations, of beauty, of frustration and deliciously tantalizing eroticism. Vietnam is a wonderland that has been flowering, recently, thanks to the relaxation of moral policing in some cities, and yet it can sometimes be repressed and tricky (especially in former North Vietnam). If you try a variety of places, you are likely to end up with a handful of fabulous experiences — not necessarily to do with massage, but with the eroticism that Western massage has lost or made mechanical, but that a few Asian countries have thankfully kept alive.

SINGAPORE MASSAGE: In my limited experience (around four visits lasting a total of 10-12 days), Singapore has a very enlightened policy towards sexual pleasure and massage (Big Brother actually *wants* people to be sexually fulfilled), and even the masseuses in hotels, who are mostly Indonesian women (among the most sensual women in the world) or sometimes Chinese, will give you an excellent professional massage, until towards the end, when the sensual dimension increases, signaling that they will essentially accommodate your needs, within reason. Prices, though higher than most other Asian countries except India, are still around half to two-thirds the price of comparable massages in the United States, and are on average, far more competent (the worst massage you'll get will be significantly better than the worst massage you'll get in the U.S.; at the top end, the competition is stiff, and the U.S. probably wins).

The Pleasures of Adultery

Often, when you've been going to the same masseuse in a Southeast Asian establishment for a while, she is seen by the other girls as your "wife." When she is away, and you ask for a different masseuse — in fact, that's the only time you can ask for a different masseuse without causing a rift and some chaos in the establishment, and a "loss of face" for the "wife" who got ditched — and you are in the room together, there is a delicious tension in the air, from both sides. It is . . . the pleasures of adultery, of an "affair." A one-time fling, which you've both been "permitted," because she is away. This can be a really exciting time, because she's going to be extra-nice to you, partly out of competitiveness and jealousy towards your "wife"; and if you are extra nice to her, you can expect something very hot to develop.

How to Have an Exciting Massage in Southeast Asia
(These are generalizations, and may not always work):

1. Choose the woman who smiles, who connects with your eyes, and who looks enthusiastic. These *could be* signals that she likes you, or that she really needs your business, and will be grateful to you for choosing her.

2. Or else, choose the woman who looks like a potentially good masseuse, but is shy, not so pretty, and is looking a bit rejected. Out of gratitude for your having chosen her, she could end up giving you a damn good massage.

3.   In Asia, remember to be soft-spoken, to smile, to be gentle, and to gracefully accept occasional setbacks; because "saving face" is such an important element of Asian society, that you do *not* want to needlessly make an enemy by being rigid about relatively trivial matters. Letting go is sometimes the best strategy. At such low prices, it is not important that you always get your way; sweetness will often take you far, and as they get to know you better, they may let their guard down and go farther than you believed possible. The offer of a little tip can often trigger enormous changes in rigid philosophical positions. This advice is the result of my having made many mistakes.

Universal Advice Directed Mostly At Customers of Western Massage

(Most of the advice that follows this paragraph applies to massages in the West, in which the average fee is $60 and up per hour.)

Negotiate Reduction For A Bad Massage

If some new form of massage that you decided to try was disappointing and unsatisfying, or if the first massage with a therapist was incompetent, negotiate down the price, because if you leave dissatisfied, the anger and betrayal, the sense of having "been taken", will lodge in your muscles and make you tenser than you were. Arrive at a compromise, some half-way point, wherein you can say, "I am paying more than I think the massage is worth, but less than what you would have liked to get for it, and that's because I realize there was a misunderstanding; but neither of us should have to bear the burden of the misunderstanding by ourselves."

Should You Patronize Hand-Helpers?

If your main intention is to get a massage, and not to receive sexual services, then you may find that in America and in certain other countries, the problem with most hand-helpers or

Happy Ending Engineers is that they are so used to and focused on making quick money that they are therefore not fair with the massage itself: they are more than likely to cheat on the time, and easily make an assumption that their customers are as impatient as they are to get to the all-too-brief Main Course. So, though there are some beauties in this field, it would be good to be clear in your own head about your major purpose: an erotic massage or a therapeutic massage for your muscle pains. Because if you go into a massage expecting both, you may come out of it still feeling some of the aches that you started with.

Should You Get Massaged By A Man?

I've had a fine massage from a man, at the Bally's Casino Health Club in Atlantic City. He was very strong, yet gentle, complete, and perfect. He never made me feel embarrassed or defensive or uncomfortable. I cannot say this of most other male massage therapists, whether heterosexual or gay (in fact, the gay ones are slightly better, because they have fewer internal conflicts about their identity). I am not particularly bothered about the sexual orientation of the masseur, so long as he is as good as the best female massage therapists, and so long as he doesn't make an "inappropriate move" on me.

The truth is that when I am desperate for a massage, I will accept it from anyone — even a man. But given a choice of two equally competent and problem-free therapists, or a choice between a female therapist who is only marginally less good than the man, I will prefer the woman, unless she cannot provide the strong massage I need (which should be strong, but not crushingly, bruisingly strong). My hunch is that the female will be more relaxing, more sensuous, more motherly and tender, more supporting of my identity as a man — and that her hands will be less calloused and therefore more soothing.

And, while I have suffered odd or wacky female therapists, the embarrassment is more acute should the therapist be male. One masseur who turned up at my door in Miami kept his oil bottle in a scrotal-looking pouch around his waist, and poured out drops of it onto my body every few minutes, not bothering to keep a hand on the subject (me) at all times. The symbolism of this is uncomfortably, even hilariously clear, and was confirmed when I found his hips swaying in a sort of dance as he massaged me, and when he had no problems brushing against my leaning tower of a pisser.

Best Masseuses Regionwise In America?

The best: from California, New York City, and New Hampshire, where there was a community called Earthstar. Many of the older, experienced masseuses have seen and been through nearly everything, and can distinguish the truth from the bullshit. If the goal is *massage*, the older (within reason), more experienced woman is most often the better choice. The worst massages in my experience? Upstate New York, Long Island (except possibly the upscale East End), and the American South, except Florida, where the massages can vary wildly in quality, but the good ones are quite good. I have zero experience of the Midwest; though I've visited Chicago a few times, I don't remember ever getting a massage over there.

In New York City, I am likely to choose East European, older, or Korean massages for quality, and Chinese masseuses for economy; I've also had outstanding massages from a few older American-born professionals, including a Brooklyn-resident masseuse named Francesca, but they are usually very busy, fully booked, and expensive.

Pressure, Degrees Of

I hope the industry decides to advertise four grades of pressure so that a customer can communicate which level he or she needs to the therapist. Grade Four, the kind of pressure that would be needed by a professional athlete, wrestler, or body sculptor. Grade Three to those whose bodies are in perfectly good shape, who often go to the gym or play sports. Grade Two to those with less-exercised, less than perfect bodies. Grade One to the over-fifty, the sick, and the convalescent.

Thai and Shiatsu Versus Oil or Swedish

Traditional Thai massages, which are partly a form of masseuse-assisted yoga, and partly a form of Shiatsu (Shiatsu has fewer movements and more pressure point therapy than Thai massage), and most of the deep massage therapies that aim to reach at and reduce your pain without the benefit of oil: I find they are not suited for the extremely tense, and for those whose body is not in good shape. They are fine for the reasonably healthy and tough individual who engages in regular exercise (and most Thai and Southeast Asian masseuses have strong, tough bodies). Not good for me, because the "traditional" or oil-less massage will often awaken the deep pain in me, will stir up the problem without healing it, and often leave me wanting more, and in a state of anxiety and reduced sense of wellbeing, sometimes much worse off than when I started. That is when I realize that my body is a mess, and that my body would require hours of this stuff if it is to get to some point of balance. On the other hand a good Swedish-type, Esalen, aromatherapy, or oil massage, which concentrates on a combination of stimulating circulation, pain relief, and deep tissue work with alternate doses of pleasure, touching, comforting and good old healing: it has me feeling rested, satisfied, taken care of, refreshed and a new person at the end of it. I am likely to feel drowsy at the end of a great oil massage, especially if I've had it just an hour to three hours before bed; if that's when I have had it, my sleep will likely help complete the healing, and it will quite likely be a good sleep. On the other hand, a massage more than 2 hours before bedtime might arouse me sexually, and would be a terrific prelude to a sexual encounter.

That's my prejudice against non-oil massages; they are fine, they may even be necessary and terrific for certain constitutions, but they do not include the healing, human component that I am looking for, and if I had to choose only one of the two, I would choose the oil or Swedish massage; which is what I almost always do.

Price Matters

Sliding scale massage fees are the answer, the compromise that will give masseuses a fair wage and at the same time not exclude all but the well-heeled. By all means, soak the rich; let them pay $150 or $200 for a massage. But let 50 percent of your massages be priced so as to be affordable to massage addicts and the poor.

In the above paragraph, I was speaking about independent practitioners. It is a sad and unjust state of affairs that massage has been partly taken over by corporations who pocket most of the fruits of their employees' labor. I was told by Oolah from Santa Rosa, California: the Bodega Bay Lodge pays its massage therapists $30 per hour of massage, while charging the customers $94 (including the service charge). The general payment that masseuses receive from establishments is supposedly $25, though one place gives them even less: $19.

My suggestion is that you as a customer make known your opinion that in any massage establishment, a masseuse ought to be paid at least 60% of what you paid.

The Double Massage Trick

A trick to watch out for. You have the hotel send in a masseuse, and a huge, domineering woman appears. You are too polite to express your reservations, though it may be obvious from your nervous manner. She pretends to know so much about massage that you are just to lie down and do what she says — that's a warning sign right away (humility and respect towards the customer are essential, unless you've specifically ordered a dominatrix). The masseuse starts massaging your feet and the back of your legs, and keeps on and on, at it. "Well, I have sore parts in my back and shoulders too, I want you to spend more time on them, so that's enough with the legs," you say. "I know," she replies. "But I have to do this *my way*. I have a system. The feet are very important. Just wait." And then, by the time she has arrived at your upper back and shoulders, and it is time for you to turn over, your one hour is up, and she asks if you would like an extra hour, because she hasn't finished. You are in deep doodoo, especially if you didn't want to spend more than the agreed price (the price the hotel had quoted to you), and especially not for a contemptuous, domineering masseuse such as she. And yet, you are not finished yet, and you would feel unbalanced and possibly even put your body at risk by not finishing the rest of the body. So you have been trapped and tricked.

This happened to me, and I ended up paying for two hours of asecond-rate massage in which the masseuse had poked me with long and dirt-filled fingernails for some of the time. A solution might be to tell the masseuse right before the massage starts which areas you expect her to complete within the agreed time.

However, even tricky massages such as these have enriched my experience, and have increased my appreciation for the really good masseuses, such as the masseuses of Cambodia, Thailand, and Indonesia, who give so much for so little: who are angels and ministers of grace, and who, collectively, along with their best Western sisters, deserve to be awarded the next Nobel Prize for Peace.

BOOK II

THE UNCENSORED MASSAGE
MASSAGE AND SEX IN AMERICA
AND ELSEWHERE

FROM MASSAGE TO MASSAGE BOOM BOOM

My first massage from a woman happened in a small, dark, windowless room in Long Island, New York. The lights were low, and only a thin cotton sheet separated my naked, trembling body from the beautiful, late-twentyish red-haired woman who held me in the palm of her hand.

"It is a therapeutic Swedish massage," she had said to me. "It will be forty-five dollars." I was at my sexual peak, and though I was a happily married man, we had just had our first baby, and I could not honestly claim that other women didn't turn me on.

"Sure," I had said. The therapy was working: alone and naked in a room with a lovely young woman, a room in which we could do whatever we wished, undisturbed. Her womanly odor, her tender voice coated with honey, her lush hair, and her concern for me as a human being: they filled the room, and filled my heart. It would have been unnatural if I did not have an erection; and the lovely Julia, barely a few years younger than I, would certainly notice it pretty soon, if she hadn't already.

And she did, and it did not upset her—there was something so human and sweet about her, I would discover over the course of a few months—for she continued to massage me gloriously, tenderly, in parts of my body that had not been touched for ages (yes, even a loving wife who has just become a mother understandably wants to have her sex quickly and be done with it). Luckily—I think Julia did not notice that, as a result of her heavenly ministrations, I had an ejaculation. Or, if she did notice, she treated this occurrence as something natural, as natural as saliva or sweat.

A few years and a few hundred massages later, now a near addict of massage (and also hounded by back pains and stress brought on by laptops and life itself), I found myself naked and with an erection in a New Hampshire swimming pool populated by just one other human being: a stark naked blonde. I had escaped the noise of New York for a writing break in the green and bucolic areas of New Hampshire, a land of meadows, streams, lakes, and vast vistas of green, with the White Mountains visible in the distance. And though I had a nearly insatiable libido in those days, this specific pocket rocket at the spa owed its existence to a large Mohawk-topped pussy, displayed between wide open legs, as if its owner were inviting Ra, the Sun God, to bless it. The said owner was a thirtyish woman with one glass eye (and one real one) and full and pert size 36D breasts. She seemed to alternate between reading a mass-market paperback and smiling vaguely at no one in particular as she lay back on a beach lounger, her mildly tanned and delicately oiled skin gleaming in the sun (indeed, there were only two of us out there in the swimming pool area at that time). It was an interesting tan, such as it was, for there was no awkward white patch where the bikini might have been—the tan was evenly distributed all over her body, the mark of a true and uninhibited sun worshipper democratically distributing wholesome sunshine to every square-millimeter of her skin. I tried to avert my gaze from the fulcrum of her being and direct it instead towards her glass eye, and then up at the hazy blue sky desperately trying to spot a swallow or a flock of Canadian geese to distract myself with, not wanting to emerge from the water in my embarrassingly erect state, my rocket devoid of its camouflaging pocket. But my eyes kept getting magnetically re-attracted to the Mohawk-topped treasure. For it was the first time that I had come across a naked stranger in a swimming pool, and I was a tongue-tied social klutz in those days. So it happened that my erection and that remarkable vagina were never ever introduced to each other, and each went home sun-kissed but otherwise lonely and unsatisfied, perhaps to be consoled by our respective hands.

Reflecting on that incident now, I credit my endless desire for massage in part to my insatiable yearning to be touched and loved, to be tenderly caressed, and at some secret level, to be enveloped in a sexual embrace. A yearning which initially proceeded from my pain, and later, became a frantic attempt to save my life and to survive the catastrophe.

However, for nearly ten years, beginning with that first massage in Long Island, New York, I went along with the line proclaimed by most American massage therapists: that massage and sex existed in separate, watertight compartments, that one had nothing to do with the other, and never, ever should. I received my massage on massage tables from professionals, and I received my sex at home in bed from my beautiful and talented wife. With rare exceptions, I responded scornfully and disapprovingly whenever someone tried to offer me massage and sex together in various creative, "combo" packages. (Except for one hilarious accident, which I describe in this book, it was relatively easy not to get confused. If the massage cost significantly more than forty-five to sixty dollars an hour, or if the advertisement used overly suggestive language or had illustrations of panting, semi-undressed women with a few loose buttons and parted lips, it was probably going to be something other than.) Though I was often sexually aroused during a massage, my Catholic upbringing (which was always in the background, despite my having become an agnostic) prevented me from burdening myself with unnecessary guilt, considering that I had, on the whole, a good marriage.

Excluding half a dozen mostly accidental episodes, my one and half thousand massages up until 1999 were all a hundred percent "legitimate", though a handful of these masseuses rather sensibly didn't bother with towels. But around the turn of the millennium, things began to change when something happened in my life.

It was more than that I ceased to have an official wife; I was also suddenly cut off from my children for two weeks or a month at a time, and I desperately needed comforting. From that point on, I so welcomed the company and touch of women, found it to be so deeply therapeutic to body and soul, in whatever form it was offered (and sometimes given without asking), that I reversed my moral position 180 degrees. If a woman was generous to me, unstinting in her touch and love, and sometimes going beyond that, she was not a sinner but a saint, a goddess, a gift from heaven.

When, for example, a masseuse's hands strayed under the towel to gently brush the bulb or head of my penis each time she made a downward movement over my thigh, and repeated this action twenty times, I didn't raise my hand and shout, "Objection, Ma'am!" I accepted it as a gift, as an act of comfort, as a deep handshake between our souls. And sometimes, when a gift such as this developed into something more profound, and led to a mutually pleasurable merging of body and soul, an erasure of the illusion of separateness, for anywhere between fifteen and thirty minutes—I didn't object to that either.

It still didn't happen too often, but I slowly realized that my earlier religious and fanatic insistence on Pure Unadulterated Massage was partial bullshit. For the spirit wants what it wants, or needs (and sometimes the spirit wants just spirits, and massage is beyond the thoughts of a man whose insides are drenched with distilled spirits). Therefore, no absolutist and Big-Brotherly moral code of one section of society should boot out one of the most salubrious and life-giving—and sometimes, life-saving—pleasures in other people's lives.

And as I traveled in Asia and in parts of Western Europe (Germany, for instance), and noticed the complete lack of embarrassment or a sense of sin about sex in the East Asian countries (even though they prefer to cover themselves in public, they are very accepting of sex in private), I realized that to the body, which is a purely biological organism without moral rules, an organism that is hardwired for the survival of the species, massage and boom boom are simply two points in a continuum, just as much as eating and boom boom, or politics and boom boom, or money and boom boom are. Boom boom (as the charming natives of Cambodia and some of their neighbors so delightfully and merrily term sex, pronouncing it halfway between boom boom and bum bum) is the sun around which the other planets of human life, such as politics, history, economics, spirituality, trigonometry, art, and yes, massage, revolve.

However, the relationship between massage and boom boom is more than philosophical or theoretical. It is not just that boom boom is simply the farthest and most intimate point in the continuum of touch and human connection that starts with a formal handshake and progresses past a hug, a clothed massage, a minimally clothed massage, a totally unclothed massage, a *mutually* unclothed massage, a mutually unclothed *body-to-body massage,* and then on to boom boom, which is arguably the essence of life, the alpha and the omega of existence.

In real life, if you were to conduct a sample survey of twenty thousand massage establishments the world over, you would realize that in many parts of the world, in the more relaxed and tropical, the Buddhist or Shinto-Confucian countries especially, massage and boom boom are Part I and Part II respectively of an organically connected whole experience. Part I is when the body is kneaded, awakened to life and good health, its circulation improved, its glands beginning to secrete the juices they should be secreting, its pleasure nodes buzzing. And as these variously aroused parts begin to shake off their former alienation, rebellion, or dysfunctional states and connect with each other, their synergy ignites Part II, or the most sacred and most vital act of human existence: fucking.

There's no better definition of Puritanism than H.L. Mencken's "the haunting fear that someone, somewhere may be happy," and it was certainly part of my Western upbringing. So I would often demand that I be given only massage, unadulterated even by dreams of boom boom. For every improper suggestion or indecent proposal the masseuse made, I mentally deducted five percent from my planned tip.

What a stick-in-the-mud I was then! For at some deep, secret level, all of us pine for the touch of our mothers and female relatives, which was so forthcoming and generous in our childhood, though more so, I was to notice later, in Eastern countries, where children below the age of five, sometimes bare-bottomed, are picked up and cuddled and carried and placed on laps by every woman and prepubescent girl in the vicinity, and consider it their birthright. And oh, the bathing and massage rituals. Sometimes, a woman will combine her bath with that of her child (or the child she is taking care of), and part of this ritual may involve a kind of intimacy that the child cannot hope to enjoy as it grows up. And the Inner Child never forgives, and is never reconciled, to this loss.

Thus you are always secretly and perhaps even unknown to yourself hungering for those intimate, uninhibited, and ungrudging intimacy and total and unconditional acceptance. So when you are touched tenderly by a masseuse with soft hands, you are aroused with warm feelings for the whole world, for all of humanity. And if your masseuse, the most immediate, breathing, perfumed, and throbbing representative of that humanity, is even passably attractive, your attention gradually turns to her, especially once the major zones of pain have been taken care of. The nicer she is to you, the nicer you want to be to her, and this feeling sometimes spills beyond the realm of verbal thanks or gifts of cash, goods, coupons, or white elephants. It could provoke a desire to respond in kind (in the ultimate example, to return love by making love).

Acknowledging this yearning to touch and to return affection (which was never consummated), one of my best Upstate New York masseuses, Lisa, the one who would whisper into my ear like a lover, "The massage is finished, thank you," would always give me a deep hug after I had dressed up and was about to leave.

And yet sometimes, especially when pain dominates your

mind and overpowers all other feelings and thoughts, when unbearable aches or tension are a stumbling block to daily living and to each moment, or when you don't wish to ruin a long-term professional relationship with the masseuse whose destiny and yours have intersected, you need to pretend to accept this artificial, manmade distinction between massage and sex simply to avoid being preyed upon for large amounts of cash or being cheated of the therapeutic massage your muscles need. Many a time has a lazy or incompetent masseuse tried to milk me (of my money) by offering a quick sexual climax, often of the hand-assisted variety (and sometimes of the orally assisted variety), hoping thus to escape the hard work that a full therapeutic massage is. (And as for escaping the real work of a massage, there are often so-called licensed massage therapists in the U.S. who will try to do this: by asking you to breathe, for example.) Rarely, and in my post-marital years, when the formerly therapeutic relationship progressed into mutually enjoyable sex, the therapeutic portion deteriorated and shrunk until I was forced to start a long and often painful search for a new masseuse: and to firmly spell out that what I was looking for was "massage *no* boom boom"—the only unambiguous term that the local taxi drivers, bellboys, guides, and touts in Southeast Asia clearly understood: a term that left them little wiggle room for their tricks and surprises.

But trying to keep the massage nonsexual or not openly erotic is easier in certain countries and cultures than in others, and indeed may be easier for Western societies that, like Bill Clinton, are able to rigidly and effortlessly compartmentalize emotions, sex, and work. True, in Thailand, a culture of therapeutic traditional Thai massage attached to students, temples, massage teachers, and massage schools exists quite apart from the world of sex—or at least as far apart as medicine and banking. Respectable family men and women, mothers, fathers, and grandmothers, get themselves massaged, sometimes in Buddhist temples, or in establishments attached to temples, sometimes in their homes, sometimes on the beach on a blanket or sheet, and sometimes in a studio or a salon on tables or mats, sometimes separated by screens. These traditional Thai massages are mostly conducted clothed, or in loose pajama-like pants and top provided by the establishment, and are 100 percent legitimate (as most prudish Westerners would term them), and are often very cheap—though in private studios and salons they can sometimes get illegitimate and sensual to accommodate your desires, usually for a hefty yet reasonable extra fee.

But in other countries, it is relatively harder to find massage that is purely and nothing but massage. You may discover that the massage you are paying for is a teasing massage designed to make you a horny wreck begging for boom boom or one of its abbreviated relatives; the Thais are masters at this, and the late-arriving Chinese, for whom 60 years of often brutal and godless Communism have left them with few religious or moral scruples, are more than a match for them, or so I have heard from tourists returning from the Chinese towns around Shenzen. In a few cases, it is organically and officially "massage boom boom"—a package deal, take it or leave it, and the *only* item on the menu. In the latter case, whether or not you take advantage of the boom boom, that's your choice, you're still paying the same or just a tiny bit less. At some point you may start to feel silly, if not totally insane, not to try a bit of what is on offer, especially if the masseuse seems willing and eager to join you in bed. Far more likely, your aroused loins or your offended ego will do the thinking for you (*What's wrong with you?* the laughing and sometimes aroused women will ask, for they too sometimes desire to have a man in their arms and wouldn't like to leave an attractive prospect untended. They will continue, provocatively: "*What, can't get it up?* No have *power?*").

Massage in this part of the world is an aphrodisiac aid to boom boom, a preparation and a provocation for boom boom, the ultimate assertion and expression of life, love and health. I imagine this un-compartmentalized view comes from an earlier and less moralistic time, when kings and princes, faced with a revolt from their underfucked multiple wives, had to be massaged so they could perform again and again, and the prestige, virility, and stability of the kingdom ensured, its populace sleeping soundly in the assurance that the Royal Member was a Member in Good Standing. And why should I, with my Western indoctrination, condemn these cultures as decadent or inferior for this reason?

It is this journey, from innocence to experience, from a naïve acceptance of my brainwashing by didactic American massage therapists to a gradual understanding of my body and the perspectives and practices of massage therapists in less stuck-up parts of the world that I wish to record here, and in the other book (*The Uncensored Massage: Thailand, Indonesia, Vietnam, China*) which delves into my Oriental massage experiences in somewhat more detail. For it is a rich journey: my over three thousand massages were received in over twenty countries around the world, from Canada to the Czech Republic, from Thailand to Scotland. What's more, I may have seen the only three-nippled masseuse in the world; she showed me her special endowment after only our second session. What it was in me that sparked this special kindness, this intimate sharing, I shall never know, though I do admit trying in a few Asian countries to pick up a bit of the local languages. And as I spoke to them like a fellow human being, an equal who was concerned, interested, warm, and grateful for their generous touch, they unlocked to me their secrets, one 39-year-old masseuse suddenly asking me if I could find her a boy friend.

This journey also includes dozens of real and warm individuals such as Elisa, of Long Island: the thing that excites me is that she, a large Romanian who is the furthest possible thing from a romantic prospect because of her plump size and looks and age, is like a mother, with me as her baby. She is like one of those Eastern mothers who are so full of love for their babies that they will kiss and wash every part, every extension, every nook and cranny, as if it were all equally sacred and divine and precious. While they massage you, they own you totally; nothing at all, no inhibition or legal code or provision of New York State Law, holds them back. How can I deny the joy of this: of being in my mid-forties, and going back, for a moment, to those blissful few months when I was a baby and completely and unconditionally loved?

That is at least part of the reason why people need massages: they want to feel cared for, touched, babied, accepted and loved unconditionally; they are looking for refuge from the harsh, unfeeling, uncaring, judging, and restrictive world, a world of boundaries fenced with legal barbed wire. God bless these women, and may many more Elisas bloom!

Not just babied, but bathed. One of the most delightful experiences you will ever have, one that is included in the price of some Eastern massages, is being soaped, bathed, and toweled dry by your masseuse. In some establishments, as in one Indian outfit a few years back, it includes just the act of soaping the unreachable parts of your back (one young masseuse named Rosie soaped my front too, but started laughing when she observed the expansive effects, and so did I, rather sheepishly). Which, back or front, is a lot better than nothing—as if any woman can trust us inept and gauche men to take proper care of ourselves! Though, reflecting on this experience later, I realized the ritual may partly have to do with the masseuses' aesthetic desire not to have to massage a smelly customer.

Also, I have fallen mildly in love with nearly every massage therapist who was good and tender on the table (and therefore, I can almost guarantee, good in bed). Though, the more beautiful the massage therapist, the stronger and more passionate the feeling, it has often happened with those who were not primarily pretty in their external appearance, but regal and symphonic in their internal and emotional selves. For a great massage is an act of love, tender, and caring, as with the lovely brown-haired Lisa from upstate New York, who has the face, hairstyle, and build of a Greek goddess, and who starts softly, her butter-soft hands spreading oil all over my body, and ends by whispering into my ear "Thank you"—so as not to rudely awaken me. It simply can't be helped; tenderness provokes my fantasy, my loving gratitude.

A good example of this generosity: At the Pennsylvania

hotel, New York, there is a warm and spacious Korean massage place where everyone is required to use the sauna and shower before a massage: an effective device, among Japanese and Korean establishments, to ensure that the customers are clean and fresh as babies before the massage. This device allows the masseuses to touch you in secret places without any reservations. My masseuse is a Korean who seems to be in her mid-forties, and who turns out to be Christian. What gentleness, softness. Of course at one point without provocation or warning she lifts up my towel and offers a compliment that Dale Carnegie would have approved of. Then, without a cue from me, she starts to kiss, lick, and suck my nipple and brush her soft hair against my chest while another hand, without the slightest warning, seeks my anus, and a finger whirls about a bit over there. I am surprised and don't know what to do, and am sure I will explode in about sixty seconds, so I exclaim "No, no, stop!"—and she stops, saying, "You are a gentleman!" And I laugh, only a semi-hollow laugh. For I am a gentleman indeed, harharhar. Well, okay, that's one of my personas (damn!), one of my multiple personalities, but why only acknowledge one?

And then she asks me how many wives I have. Twenty, I say. How about twenty-one, she asks. And to each direction I give her— "Massage here more please"—she replies, Thank you. She's singing along with the classical muzak oozing from the walls, and stops to ask, "Can I sing for you?" She doesn't grudge me her femininity, her intimacy, her motherhood. She is too gentle for me to grudge her my high-end tip. For I get a feeling that with each such new soul I meet, that I am enriched, that it is my good fortune to have met her. And let's face it: there are not that many of them left, in this increasingly commercial world. A B-minus rating for the massage, an A-plus rating for her demeanor and humanity.

Indeed, I have had as many different massages as I have had masseuses, because every person brings their special mix of personality, training, and temperament to the massage, and these massages have drained my pockets of thousands of dollars, but at least now I have a book: the uncensored confessions of a massage addict, as true and unwhitewashed as James Joyce would have brought you from the deepest recesses of Bloom's blooming brain and Molly's bloomers. And though there are thousands of massage establishments the world over who have a strict policy of massage *no* boom boom— sometimes not the most ideal or intelligent state of affairs—I am thankful even for them (and especially for them), because a world with not enough boom boom would be a much harsher and less bearable place if there was no massage either.

And I think: Instead of airdropping bombs and Special Forces and Navy Seals on the terrorist-infested areas of the world, thus infuriating the innocent locals by blasting wedding parties to tiny shreds of flesh and hanks of hair and bone— thus breeding more terrorists and recruits for Al Qaeda hell-bent on avenging their vaporized relatives—George W. Bush ought to have dropped Special Masseuse Forces, possibly nicknamed the Pink Berets, on Afghanistan. What a superb massage by a caring, loving woman does is not just drain you of your tension, but drain you of your anger and your accumulated resentments towards the world and even sometimes of a sense of purpose (a bit like the effects of marijuana, which I have too little experience with, except for a few Jamaican brownies and Cambodian "Happy" Pizzas). Just before the massage, you may have decided you were going to make the Olympics Swimming Team, become a billionaire, reinvent the wheel, design a better mousetrap, or conquer the world by the age of 25. After a gloriously relaxing massage, you just want to sleep: whether alone, or with a woman. Your ambitions don't seem as important, indeed they don't seem to have any point, for you have become overcome by a feeling of peace and oneness towards the world. So the Al Qaeda terrorist will miss boarding the plane he had planned to hijack and smash into a landmark building, and the suicide bomber will say to himself, "Well, maybe I am still ready to do the deed, but I would first like to enjoy a few more of these massages that I have been missing all my life. Heaven and the promised seventy-two buxom virgins can wait just a while longer." Consider how, with a bit of kindness and understanding, a handful of masseuses might have changed history and saved hundreds of thousands of innocent lives?

The massages I describe in this book are mostly about touch, acceptance, and tender loving care that occasionally spills over into sex. They are most often about pain, and sometimes about sore muscles and large swaths of neglected epidermis seeking their share of attention, fondling, mothering, or tender loving care, because most of the time, we are stomachists and penisists and mindists: we vastly favor these three organs, while neglecting the rest of our bodies. For example the underside of the forearm, the back of the knees, the inner thighs, and even the armpits, whose only interest for most people is that they be washed and deodorized: it's almost as if they are pariahs in the caste hierarchy of body parts. In a massage, which is anatomical democracy in action—or should be—they are collecting their democratic due, or at least a portion of their due, for a good massage makes sure that no part of the body is left untouched. Bar none, except, perhaps, the staff of life and its two supporting actors.

This book also examines the philosophical issues and practical issues behind massage, and includes issues of global significance as the Guantanamoing of penises, undercover emissions, the Zen of Balls, the global sexual famine, and how a good masseuse could save your life.

NO-PANTS MASSAGES IN AMERICA

In a middle-class neighborhood of Manhattan close to the entrance of the Midtown Tunnel and filled with monotonous brownstone apartment buildings, I met my second American masseuse, 35-ish, darkhaired, and operating out of a studio that was also her home. Not only didn't offer me a towel, but simply said, "Take off *all* your clothes and lie on the table"— pointing to the center of the room.

Around this time, we rented a home in the Long Island suburbs, but I still regularly visited Manhattan for theatre, art movies at the Film Forum and Lincoln Center, bookstores, readings, and the hipster, young and artistic atmosphere of Greenwich Village, the East Village and Soho. Now I had an additional reason for my Manhattan visits: massage, which was fifty times more easily available, and with far greater diversity and professional quality, than in dull, suburban Long Island. Janet had ten years of experience, a Siamese cat, and an apartment strewn with cat hair and cat toys. A painted portrait of her younger self showed that she had once been quite a beauty, though now she seemed a bit stressed. She was dressed in a jeans jacket that allowed a view of ample cleavage, and tight faded jeans that emphasized her butt and cut into her pussy, making a camel's toe of it.

I proceeded to undress as directed, though I had such an instant erection, the result of my excitement at this novel experience, that I had difficulty wriggling out of my tight jeans. When I did, I lay on the table nude with a monstrous erection whose existence she seemed to take no notice of. It was a novel and puzzling experience: to have a woman observe my aroused naked body, my pole pointing at the sky, and not seem to feel, think, or say a thing. So each time I would think of getting a massage from her—I could be at my home, or on the train from Long Island to the city—I would have an erection or a trouser smile that would last at least for a few minutes until something else, say the gruff voice of a ticket collector, distracted my thoughts.

Janet would apply oil to and massage every part of me except the sex organs themselves, and her massages had a completeness that those with excessive hang-ups could not give. If a masseuse was good, I didn't care if she covered me with ten blankets, so long as I could still breathe and when the time came, she attended to each and every part that needed therapeutic attention (excepting the Big One and his little twin brothers). But once I got used to Janet's open-air policy, any incompetent masseuse enforcing modesty with a heavy hand would leave me feeling cheated.

It also helped that Janet really liked my friends A. Ductor and G. Luteus Maxim (US)—who happen, coincidentally, to be friends of Al Gore too, if his accuser Molly is to be believed. (Meaning, Janet spent a considerable length of time massaging my and Al Gore's favorite muscles: the adductor muscles (inner thighs) and the gluteus maximus muscles (butt, ass, buttocks, bottom cheeks—take your pick, but leave *my* butt alone!). Favorite, because they were both highly sensuous highly ache-filled areas for me. You can use your imagination to guess what happened, or else I'll tell you later in the book.

However, as I was blessed with a lovely wife and loving children—though that didn't stop me from lusting in my heart after Manhattan's legions of lovely women, and freely admitting it in my writings—my massages, having begun in Therapeutic Wholeness and in Medical Necessity, remained thus; for many years, I was sanctimonious about the completely "therapeutic" nature of the massage I wanted.

But after ten years of wholesome and pure massage, I ran into a Russian immigrant masseuse named Ella, a young mother who was sweet, warm, quite pretty, and besides earthy—the kind who makes your sanctimoniousness melt away in about thirty seconds. While massaging me, she noticed that I had a boner which had made a tent of the brief towel, and that was causing me stress because of my unsuccessful attempt to hide it. She asked if she could "take care" of it for me. With automatic and pompous sanctimoniousness I said "No, I prefer to keep my massage within the realm of therapeutic relaxation, and to have my erotic needs attended to by my wife." Said she: "There's no way this massage is going to relax you so long as you have that." I saw her point, and the absurdity of my rigid stand (and also of my rigid cockstand); it was as if a 1000-watt light bulb had suddenly lit up in my brain. And most of all, I appreciated her concern and her naturalness, and began to realize that the word "therapeutic" need not be restricted to just certain parts of the body. That even the body believes in equality and equal rights, and despises discrimination between its various parts.

I now believe that in some cases, helping a male client ejaculate may be an essential part of the massage process, because any bottled up sexual tension inhibits the very relaxation the massage is designed to effect. But I also equally support the right of the masseuse to choose *not* to do it. Besides which—full disclosure here—I myself almost never ask for it or even *allow* it, surrendering only very rarely to almost-Godfather-like offers I cannot refuse. Why?

Partly because my surplus mojo would sometimes burst through the emergency door and leak out without any specific intervention and sometimes without my even wanting it. But also partly because an extortionate mindset often takes over many masseuses the moment they think they have an erect penis and its owner as their prisoner. In certain Asian countries, for just the work of five minutes it takes her to make you ejaculate, a masseuse might demand double or triple the price of the massage itself. Because she has you by the balls, to speak metaphorically (and with some Thai masseuses, literally so, for they don't believe in using light artillery when they can bring in the heavy artillery right away and achieve their objective—try arguing with someone who is in a position of such advantage!). And this "tip" goes entirely into her pocket. (There are other reasons for my usually declining a so-called happy ending, which I will explain later.)

After meeting Ella, however, I gradually gave up my humorless moral objections and self-duping mind games. And when I found a masseuse who was affectionate towards me, relaxed, and not extortionate, I relaxed my own attitude. As with Kristina, a masseuse who was so comfortable and relaxed with my body and with me that she spread my legs one foot apart, and massaged almost every place she could find between them with perfect ease and naturalness and love, and then turned me around and picked up my penis without my permission, as if she owned it, as if she had every goddamn right in the world. I was so surprised and grateful by then for the trust implied in this gesture that I let her do what she was going to do, what she almost *wanted* to do. By now, I had discovered that life and love were fragile things, and that life was too short for me to affect a holier-than-thou attitude and say, "No, I don't want *pleasure*. I am nobler than that. I want only a *massage*, thank you!"

Or the plump Romanian masseuse Elisa, who I rate a 9 on 10. If there's one masseuse every massage therapist should experience simply to know what the competition is like, she should try Elisa. (In fact, a masseuse who doesn't scope the competition is a dumb masseuse). She goes straight for your tits. Hers is that perfect combination of pleasure, therapeutic relief, nurturing, erotic ecstasy, teasing and frustration, and innocence; she is the perfect counterargument to anyone who argues that masseuses are just of two types: legitimate and illegitimate. Hers is the eroticism of the unknown, the mysterious, the ambiguous, and the unexpected.

Her soft fingers graze your perineum when they travel up your thighs, and no matter what she's doing when she's engaged with the middle four-fifths of your body, she is brushing up against your rampant or slightly subdued penis. Her fingers are soft, her face is a combination of mischief and childish playfulness. "Who, me?" her expression seems to say, as she accidentally—oops, sorry!—squeezes the joy juice out of you.

I met Elisa around 1998, when my marriage was unraveling, and the extra stress needed extra comforting. However, I will also admit that in my earlier, pompously Righteous and Holier-than-Thou years, there were two accidents.

The first was with Janet, my regular masseuse for twelve years. On my second visit, without even asking me, she applied some oil to her hands and, before I realized what was happening, picked up my cock—which had been erect throughout the massage—and started moving her hands up and down on it. This was so new for me, it being years before I would hear of lingam massage (the sophisticated cousin of the lowly dick massage), that I didn't object, but just watched in fascination, as if hypnotized. And as I had already been aroused for a full hour, it didn't take me too long to come.

However, Janet was so mechanical and clinical that I regarded hers as a purely medical intervention, and an artist's experiment in the pursuit of his art ("try everything once"). But as I was morally ambivalent about this and didn't tip her, or even say "Thanks for lending a helping hand to my Little Monster," the "accident" was never repeated.

The second accident happened at a semi-upscale Murray Hill joint catering to a yuppie and hedonistic *New York Magazine* clientele. Janet being busy that day, I was desperately calling up phone numbers from *The Village Voice* and then from *New York* magazine, and discovered one place that had an immediate opening at 2 pm.

At this well-decorated spa with plants and a fish tank, I was shown to a room and asked to strip fully, lie on the table face up, and await my masseuse.

I did as told, and as there was no towel, and the mystery of who my masseuse might be excited me, I was fully erect even before anyone had even touched me. Then a gorgeous young mulatto woman, either Caribbean or Brazilian, perhaps 22, with a sweet smiling face and a spectacular body, came in, saw what was on the table, and decided to seize the day (had she watched movie *Seize The Day?* I wondered later). She slipped out of her clothes within seconds and, with not a word exchanged, easily and expertly, with her juicy and nearly hairless vagina, mounted my fully perpendicular tool! I was astonished, for it was like a goddess descending from the heavens in answer to my prayers—too stunned to say anything, and too ecstatic at my luck to register my procedural or philosophical objection (or perhaps I had been sedated by the tranquilizers I was then taking). Squatting over me, she slid up and down, and up and down, smooth as a pole dancer, and with a mix of such tenderness, enthusiasm, and pure lust that, it being one of my rare extramarital experiences as well as perhaps my only extramarital woman-on-top experience, I might have ejaculated quickly; however, I was only 40 years old or so then, virile and in great physical shape, having recently sired three sons one after another, and had this biological quirk that in the mornings and afternoons, unlike evenings and nights, it could sometimes take me forever to come, even to the point of frustration; so I wasn't about to ejaculate quickly.

But just five minutes into this dream, a female supervisor burst into the room, observed the proceedings with shock, and exclaimed, "No, no! Not *him!*" And instantly, my mulatto lover climbed off my disappointed pole and with a shy smile, hurried into her clothes and out of the room.

Then, slowly, I got it. Besides giving regular massages, this place was also a cover for a high class brothel, and I was not to be fucked, because I hadn't paid for sex. I was paying seventy dollars for the hour, and not even in your wildest fantasies could you have sex with a beautiful young woman in New York

City for less than double that figure, if not quadruple.

I now guess my accidental lover had been a newcomer, and recall with nostalgia that innocent time when one could still think of fucking without a condom—I mean, the AIDS scare had gotten around quite a bit, but some of us still believed that the disease struck mainly gays and drug addicts, and were willing to take our chances. But wait a moment, stop! The AIDS issue is a pure afterthought—a retrospective comment inserted as I write this many years later. At that particular moment, I was in a dream; as in a terrific sexual dream which you simply don't want to end, one of those dreams in which even though you half-know it is a dream, you are still moving your hips and hoping that it will somehow continue and perhaps even become real. So all I did was lie there passively watching her slide up and down my cock with the lithe grace of a dancer while my heart thumped with joy. The morbid fear of disease is a luxury of the Super-Haves, of the Elliot Spitzers and the Donald Trumps (though not of the multiple-bareback-riding Tiger Woodses, admittedly), not of someone for whom it was the first such occurrence.

Given the magnitude of my loss (my cosmic but subsonic shout, "Oh, Shit!" was recorded in a faraway galaxy), my memory has deleted what exactly happened after that (my guess is they sent in a substitute to give me a regular massage); because in those days, as I was still married, and mainly quite happily too, I had to write these truly rare incidents down in a secret diary and hope they wouldn't be discovered. What else was I going to do: sobbingly confess to my still most beloved and precious wife that for a few heavenly minutes I had been the victim of an ambush, of a vicious assault by a suddenly descending and gorgeous vagina?

THE WALL STREET TANTRIC MASSAGE
AND THE NUDE FINNISH PUSSYCAT

Manhattan, the capital of the world, a city packed with the top talents in every field, from neurosurgery to bondage, and from literature to gastronomy, is also home to some awful pretenders and snake oil salesmen; this capital of the world also attracts world class con men and women, some of whom pass themselves off as spiritual leaders and healers and advertise their incredible offerings to the credulous in *The Whole Life Times* or some such organ.

Ah, yes. It is an age in which any two-bit twerp who recently operated a hot dog stand in a corn-pone town thinks that by holding his or her hands in the air above some pathetic sucker and saying "Breathe deeply" or "Feel the spirit!" he is transformed into a *healer*. A healer, and therefore a (Cabinet) Minister of Universal Energy who must be paid with reverence and universally acceptable hard cash (they don't mind if you go easy on the reverence, but the hard cash is non-negotiable). And everyone who comes to these healers is, by definition, sick, guilty, inferior, a retard who must be condescended to and told things like, "You may keep your underwear on" (and sometimes, "you may keep your radiation-proof body suit on").

But one adventurous afternoon in the late Nineties—by now, my published novel had received considerable acclaim and I felt more confident—I boarded a train to Penn Station and then the subway to Wall Street and emerged into a street that was a canyon in the skyscraper section of downtown New York, and not far from the Twin Towers. I entered one of these skyscrapers, and went in for an experience that had all the hallmarks of the good old-fashioned American sucker story. And yet, it had enough novelty, mystery, open-mindedness, and excitement for me as to justify at least a portion of the hundred bucks I shelled out.

It was a "Tantric Massage" administered by a Russian woman and man, between 29 and 35, both looking immensely sharp, like KGB double agents, this being a time when post-Soviet Russians had invaded New York City and were buying up real estate, spas, and hair salons. The setting: a Wall Street office room decorated with the pictures of an Indian guru facing a Christian Cross, these antithetical artifacts surrounded by candles and a chalice, incense sticks spreading a sandalwood perfume through the room's heated air. After undressing behind a partition, I was instructed to enter the room naked, which I did, preceded by my full-mast flagpole, and watched by two pairs of eyes. As directed, I lay down on a mattress laid on the floor, and was subjected to a synchronized massage by a pair of female hands on my left side and a pair of male hands on my right. My male chauvinist consciousness tried to concentrate on the soft female half of the touch (and the fact that she, Yippie!, briefly brushed her finger against my pee-pee). The so-called tantric massage ended with a "prostate massage"—a massage of dick, balls, and perineum simultaneously—which, finally, made me ejaculate in full view, as the Tantrics had desired (and why would I wish to disappoint them?). It was my most spiritual and public coming ever, and I wonder now if there was a secret camera recording these proceedings for history or for prying eyes—and if so, if I could buy the rights to the film.

Anyway, once I had cleaned myself up and dressed up, I was allowed to ask questions of The Master. I could say the name of a woman, and I would be told what kind of sexual relations I could expect with her. Having just had an emission, thanks mainly to the woman's probing fingers, I was a little dazed; my memory cells were out in the streets partying and celebrating my good luck.

When you think about it (and I mustn't be too unkind, for I don't quite know the relative percentages of their actual knowledge and charlatanry), it was hilarious: the author of a well-known, sexually liberated book receiving sexual advice from a pair of charlatans. Still, I didn't want to miss out on some fun, especially as I had paid for it, and as a writer has a certain license in these things. He can pretend and probe and go with the flow, because ultimately he'll turn every damn thing, every big shit and small, into literary material.

I said, "Luba"

"Oh, a Russian girl? Well, she hasn't had much good sex in her life, so what she needs is not sensitivity, but hard fucking. A good strong dick. She could potentially really go for you."

I said, "Sheila."

"Sheila, she is good, but she has another man that she might be interested in."

What about my sexual future?

"You will reach your peak in 2-3 years. Then you will have lots of women and pleasure. At 51, you will start losing interest in physical sex; women will come to you more for play and fun than for your fucking."

Am I average or above average? I asked.

"You are well above average. And if you only do the exercises contracting your prostate without tensing your buttocks and legs, you'll be able to control the length of your erection tremendously.

"Sex is very important to you. You think a lot about it. It is okay to think about it, but don't worry about it, and it will come to you. *Women, they need to feel that you are cool and relaxed. They can sense tension and worry. If you are relaxed, they'll come to you.*"

I had to admit that these sounded like words of wisdom, besides which in three out of four specific answers to my questions, his judgment had been uncannily accurate. *To have the relaxed attitude to life.* That itself was worth perhaps 500 bucks, or five times what I had paid. Though, despite his prediction, I am still interested in sex, and though considerably more experienced, cannot quite claim that I have had to fight back legions of women. Though, to speak in their defense, they were probably waiting for me to have the relaxed attitude to life.

* * *

Immigrants, the lifeblood of America, and the chief reason for its vitality, creativity, and continuous reinvention of itself, had begun to revitalize New York's massage scene in the Nineties. While Russians entered it in the early Nineties, their hallmarks being technical proficiency, nonchalance about naked bodies, and giving a decent butt massage, the Koreans entering in the latter half were juicy Lucys, often arousing the men until they begged for some relief. And while stray Koreans like Jeannie could be extremely good, Korean masseuses were generally more expensive and expected large tips, so I only used them when my regular masseuses were unavailable.

It's a horrid, gray and drizzly late Autumn day in Manhattan, a day in which one massage appointment after another turns bad. And then, suddenly, it turns out that these rejections were the best thing to happen to me. For the next number I called yielded a warm "Yes, I can give you an appointment right now." And 20 minutes later, I meet the most glorious Finnish woman I have ever met and spend the best eight-five dollars I have ever spent in my life.

Her name, she tells me, is Tessa. She is around 5'9", but looks taller, because she wears high heels. She has light blonde hair.

The room is lit with candles and a soft table lamp, and perfumed by incense. To my surprise, she asks me to get naked.

"Not many people come in here as horny as you," she says, smiling, as I drop my pants, revealing a flagpole at a 90 degree angle to my legs.

Her sweet nature matches her voice on the phone; what's

more, to my surprise, she strips and performs the massage in the buff, with not even a toe-ring or a bracelet on her. The vision will stay with me forever: of glorious, pert, pink-nippled breasts and a pussy with only a faint fuzz of golden hair—a curvaceous body to die for. The face of a goddess: high cheekbones, blue eyes, blond hair, classic beauty. Like a *Playboy* centerfold, like one of the women from the movie *Caligula.*

Is it a dream? She even spreads her pussy's lips to show me her inner sanctum—those ruby-colored inner lips. It is absolutely weird, the architecture of the moment: to be domed, not by the Sistine Chapel ceiling, but by a glorious golden pussy, so to speak. And, surprise, surprise! She feels not an ounce of shame about exposing her body thus.

She also lets her well-oiled breasts trace circles of various parabolic shapes on my chest and belly clockwise, then anticlockwise.

The variety of techniques surprises me. Rubbing her breasts against various parts of my body, drawing her hair over my back and buttocks, making every pore come tinglingly alive; applying oil to her breasts, then massaging my penis with them.Having her hair graze different parts of my body.

At one point, while her mouth was occupied with delivering doses of ecstasy to my lower half, her vulva was directly above my face, and it looked so clean, golden, and delicious, and her body emitted such a rapturous scent, that my multilingual tongue, almost as if it had a mind of its own, leaped out of my mouth and started to lick the butter-soft lips dangling above me, like grapes at some Roman orgy—one of the few times I have ever licked anyone's cunt—and was rewarded with pure vaginal nectar.

At one point, she cradled each of my hands and then each of my feet in the cavity of her vulva while she was busy massaging the upper part of my leg or arm . . . I can't believe my luck: all I had expected was a competent massage.

So what's the catch?

It seems there's none. She is just a genuinely nice and sensual person from one of the freest countries in the world.

Maybe I will write her story, I say to her, effusively. Her massage is completely unimportant to me; she is. My dormant romantic, passionate self has been aroused.

I ask her when she came to America.

Six weeks back, she replies.

"That explains it," I say."I hope you don't change."

In a moment of wild fantasy, I think I ought to try to get this Finnish masseuse for myself before someone else gets her, or before she loses what is fresh and original about her. I am even willing to go to Finland along with her and get lost in there. No, why complicate things? I'll try to meet her after the massage and to make her my lover.

I am exultant, I feel different.

"Where have you been all my life?" I blurt out—a phrase I have never, ever before uttered in real life, being merely a corny line I heard in some movie! And now it just bursts out of me, spontaneously.

After the massage, Tessa treats me with special kindness and respect for my being a writer, a published author—a special quality I noticed in the Russians, Czechs, and Finns I met at the time, most of whom were well-read, and had a pretty much universal and profound reverence for writers, and who were less likely to respond with dispiriting comments such as, "A writer? Oh. Written any bestsellers?" or "I have an idea for a book; will you write it for me?"

She also tells me later that there could be no actual sex, for she had a boy friend. Smitten and greedily hoping to graduate to real sex, I made the mistake of telling her I loved her.

Later, I realized that it was more that in the sexual intimacy we had reached, and in the rapture I felt at the sweetness of her person, I felt something like love for her—a love mingled with gratitude and awe. But I didn't explain all this, and said simply, "I love you"—as if this might earn me a promotion to fourth base.

Bad move. For she was one of those literal women who responded that since she had a boy friend, and as I had used the word love, she couldn't see me anymore. To think that my only experience until then with someone with the exquisite body of a blonde Penthouse Centerfold, fully waxed or naturally hair-disadvantaged, with a generously large and swollen-lipped, silky smooth, vulva: and I had blown it?

Later, I understood her highly liberal, yet compartmentalized thought process: she had promised her boy friend that she would be selling erotic services, but not love. Eroticism, pure and unadulterated, had been distilled from the rather viscous mix that it is part of, in real life; and this pure eroticism could be marketed in capitalistic McBites or occasional Whoppers, with a little philanthropically minded erotic service to humanity thrown in. I am flattered that she thought my love real enough—and I wondered if she perhaps felt some herself too.

Meanwhile, there would be no other massage in this erotic league until I began my post-divorce visits to Southeast Asia.

HOW A MASSEUSE MAY SAVE YOUR LIFE

In a Filipino town not far from Manila, in a massage shop tucked away amidst the clatter of jeepneys, traffic, and loud music coming out of assorted shops, it was 26-ish Rea, who has the broad benevolent face of a Buddha, and is always generous and unstinting with her shy but broad and heartfelt smiles, like sunshine breaking through the clouds . . . it was Rea who finally brought home to me how a truly good masseuse may end up saving your life.

I have for some years now been having around one hundred fifty massages a year, which is possible and affordable in certain countries of Asia where labor is cheap (even in India, if you are able to directly connect with and make a regular arrangement with a masseuse, bypassing bloodsucking intermediaries who in some Asian countries cheat masseuses of most of their income).

And yet it was Rea who became the first masseuse in some months to touch my groin, to touch it feelingly, and to discover a bump there—what could be a cyst or a tumor. It was something the others hadn't noticed, even though they may have touched me there. It was something even my lovers hadn't noticed (bad, bad girls!).

And why did Rea find this bump while the others didn't?

Because she has such a pure mind, the issues of sex or modesty simply don't enter her head. The others lack the Zen quality of being in the moment, of being at every moment fully and one hundred percent occupied with the thing that they are doing, and nothing else. Even while massaging you, they may be chatting with the masseuse in the next cubicle perhaps, or listening to music, or perhaps to the music in their head, remembering some argument they had with a boy friend, or complimenting themselves on their rote-like technique, while forgetting to concentrate on the person on the table and the specific contours and vibrations emanating from the part they are working on.

Whereas, when Rea is feeling your body, she is also *feeling for* your body. Her compassion is nurturing, like a concerned and loving mother's, and she was able to zero in on something wrong that even I had missed, because even I don't go thoroughly over all the parts of my body palpating each separate square inch to see where something might be amiss. When I am in the shower, I am hurriedly soaping myself and trying to get done with this unavoidable but not necessarily ecstatic task as quickly as possible, and just making broad moves with my hands to get the soap on and then off, trying to handle large swaths of flesh in one stroke.

As for doctors these days: doctors are afraid even to shake your hand. Even with their sensation-deadening gloves on, their hands race over your body, only examining the spots that *you* point out to them. This is quite unlike Rea, who owns your body while she is massaging it; once you have implicitly given her your permission by showing her your trust, she checks it thoroughly.

Not spouses. Spouses may simply go for the main parts: the attractive parts of your body, your Venices and Taj Mahals and Eiffel Towers, while leaving out the Rwandas and Chads and Three Mile Canals, areas that are hidden or not easily within reach in the normal face-to-face coupling positions (which itself may be a good reason to engage in sixty-nine and other bizarrely angled Kama Sutra positions, including the standing on one's head position, every now and then, notwithstanding the inconvenience or the risk of bursting into laughter and losing your erection).

And so, your masseuse may one day save your life. In addition to delivering not negligible daily benefits such as boosting your immunity, giving you stress relief (yes, stress kills), and making you feel more human. But only if the masseuse is good, caring, and is in it for more than just the money. That is why I think this is an important book, passionately making the case not just for having technically proficient and caring massages, but for good, unobstructed, and broadminded massages, and also for the exchange of massages between couples: a one-week course in "How to Massage Your Lover" ought to be a prerequisite for granting a marriage license or a divorce. Well, if not a prerequisite, then at least entitling one to a cash benefit.

Should there be any doubt in your mind regarding its therapeutic benefits, the highly reputed Mayo Clinic has this assurance on its website: "Brush aside any thoughts that massage is only a feel-good way to indulge or pamper yourself. To the contrary, massage can be a powerful tool to help you take charge of your health and well-being, whether you have a specific health condition or are just looking for another stress reliever.".

WHILE MY GUITAR GENTLY WEEPS

[This chapter is dedicated to one of my favorite Beatles songs, "While My Guitar Gently Weeps"]

"Everything all right?" asks Lisa, probably my best North American masseuse ever, a goddess who lived at the foot of the Catskill Mountains. Soothing and soporific New Age music is playing softly in the background of the air-conditioned room, and the lighting is about 1.5 candles bright.

"Yes," I reply.

But I am not being completely honest. I want to pour my heart out to her, who has been so good to me, but cannot. Rather, I dare not, for I am afraid the unwelcome truth will spoil everything.

At last, I am writing a book, and now will tell the naked truth, come what may.

First of all, a centering joke.

Q: Why do men have a hole in their penis?

Answer 1: So Oxygen can get to their brain. (If you are a woman, this answer is 100% correct.)

Answer 2: So the baby maker's tiny little wriggling babymakers can spurt out, hunt for an ovum, and make babies. (If you are a man, this is the only correct answer.)

And it's true. The penis and its twin co-conspirators run us men, ruling our destiny; it is all part of the program of the species.

Yet, for years and years in America, where massage occupied, in the Eighties and Nineties, a demi-religious penumbra somewhere between a medical procedure and a pilgrimage to Lourdes, I would feel guilty whenever, in the course of the massage, I was sexually aroused to the point where I had an involuntary discharge of mojo—that is, an ejaculation. The guilt would grip me regardless of (or perhaps because of) the joke I had made up many years earlier in college: *There are two kinds of sins: sins of commission, and sins of emission.* I had erections, of course, half the time during my massages; I might be slightly embarrassed by these erections, but I knew I couldn't help them, and any masseuse must know that it's an occupational hazard (or perk, if she were to see the positive side, like Mae West, who famously said, "Is that a gun in your pocket, or are you just glad to see me?"). For some men are hornier than others; and if you can't politely ignore it, at least try not to get too steamed up about it.

But unintended sudden emissions, though nearly always occurring beneath a towel and unknown to the masseuse, seemed like an incursion into the realm of illegality and trouble. Because the unwritten and unspoken understanding seemed to be: This is a therapeutic massage for pain relief, you ought *not* to be getting any kind of sexual satisfaction or relief. *Stop! It is forbidden!*

But in real life, the boundaries between massage and sexual excitement are famously porous. How can you receive warm and intimate touches from a sweet and gentle woman without getting a bit aroused—unless you're dead down there, or you are a block of stone, without an ounce of feeling? For me, my whole body was a sexual instrument: about the only non-erogenous parts of my body were my knees, elbows, hair, and fingernails, so long as soft feminine fingers did not stray into surrounding territories. But nipples and their surrounding areas, buttocks, thighs (back, front, and inner), and lower abdomen, and sometimes even the flanks of my trunk, were highly erogenous—and yet, with the exception of nipples, flanks, and lower abdomen, these were also the areas with the most muscular tension, the greatest need of massage, along with my upper back and shoulders. Whereas hands and forearms, along with the entire chest and armpits, all important areas requiring massage—were only moderately erogenous.

For years, therefore, I would sometimes have an unintended emission and keep it under my hat—metaphorically speaking. It happened with Julia (sorry, Julia), with Janet (of course she had to notice, as she provided no towel, but she said nothing), and most anxiously, with my best American masseuse, Lisa. Keeping silent, I would feel a bit embarrassed, in any case. Not because my body was behaving naturally and healthily, as it should, but because I feared Lisa's later discovery of something sticky or coagulated on her sheets and towels, and the consequent banning of me (cut off in the blossoming of my sin, I think, with melodramatic exaggeration); for she was such a fabulously good masseuse, so head and shoulders above every other masseuse for a hundred miles, I feared that like I feared death.

One day, however, I thought the secret was out. I relate it in contemporaneous words:

Lisa discovers, or must have discovered. Using a sheet instead of the usual towel today, she let her fingers stray on both sides of my left-leaning, 75-percent erect, penis, touching it twice, and ten seconds after she had left the scene, possibly to fetch a towel, I quickly cupped the glans in my hand and contained the spray within my palm. Within seconds she returns to the room, and noticing some disturbance, asks me, "Everything all right?" "Yes," I reply, desperately trying to wipe my hands off on the sheet that I am lying on, and not having the heart to tell the truth, which is: *Heck, baby, you are all I have! It's easier to find a new lover than a good massage therapist. How could I possibly tell you what really happened and risk losing you?* But the mystery remained: Did she know that this sometimes happened? Was she being secretly mischievous with her seemingly innocent question? After all, she was a natural, unperturbed, not uttering a meaningless "sorry" after having twice brushed my soft-skinned but not-soft pee pee.

Barely two days later, I am back on her massage table, and perversely, my dick gets hard at the mere thought of what happened last time, how narrow my escape, and I have no idea how this naughty thing of mine is going to behave today. Perversely, in remembrance of its performance the last time, my dick decides to punish me with a repeat.

And with me being already aroused by my *thought,* it happens again. This time I splurt into a towel, and seconds later, gosh, she just lifts the towel and takes it away, leaving me exposed but saying nothing. *Gosh, Lisa, say something! Do you know?* I cannot think of any explanation but her intrinsic kindness and charitableness. So later, I gift her an autographed copy of my novel, and she hugs me for it.

For years, I suffered this conflict in silence (who knows how much business the resulting tension gave to massage therapists), often engaging in furious mental arithmetic to distract myself (and in the process, losing some of the relaxation I had come to the massage therapist for in the first place). Finally one day, I plucked up the courage to ask an American massage therapist I had gotten comfortable with (all of these episodes had occurred in America, for that is where I am most terrified of Big Sisterly moral reprimand): "What if you have a male customer who ejaculates on the table during the massage, and you discover it later?"

"I would simply take it as something else that someone leaves on my table, like breast milk, or menstrual blood," she replied. "Most of the time, I wouldn't notice. But if I did, it would be okay for me if he didn't bring it up, and I didn't bring it up."

God, what a noble and lofty woman, such wisdom and understanding there! How I wish I had heard these very words many years back, and from at least a few massage therapists. How much agony and anxiety and self-criticism it might have saved me. But now, thinking even more radically, I think perhaps the man doesn't merely need to be tolerated, he actually *needs*, or would at least be better off with, acceptance and understanding from the woman that what has happened is okay by her; for, when she is silent, he is unsure if he has it. Or if he needs forgiveness from her, in addition to his own forgiveness, does he have that?

These pleasant and comforting episodes, with Lisa and the masseuse who articulated her enlightened position, came much later. Many years earlier, a New Orleans masseuse had chased after me on the street just to hurl the accusation, "You ejaculated!" And earlier, another masseuse had refused to massage me further because she observed a certain fluid emission. And I thought: "But I believe in the constitutional right to freedom of emission, and the right to the privacy of my emissions. I object to the policing of my emissions, which are as involuntary as breathing, and dependent on the complex and individualistic architecture of my brain cells—which not even thirty psychoanalysts working for 30 years will quite be able to unravel. It's not as if I turn around and shoot off into the masseuse's face and open mouth; mostly, I try to prevent it by distracting myself, but if the urge is unstoppable, I do it with the utmost care to avoid discovery or embarrassment, and yet, I cannot always expect that my trail-covering measures will be foolproof."

Therefore, for readers in similar conundrums, I have crafted a few other post-emission-discovery responses. To a Lomi Lomi masseuse: "Well, I suppose I just produced a few Hawaiian mini-kids. Say Aloha to them, will you? Need some Lomi-Lomi juice?" Or the simpler: "It ain't my fault, honest, I am a nice guy, but I have never been able to train my dick to think pure thoughts." On the other hand, why should I have to keep proving to others that I am a nice guy? Whew, what a burden!

Or a longer, more serious and philosophical explanation (take a deep breath): "This emission is a purely physical and automatic response like a knee jerk or a sneeze, a conditional reflex, spasmodic and involuntary. The pleasure I get from a massage is from the foreplay, so to speak, that has preceded the emission: the expectation, the sensual quality of the touch, the rhythmic movements. Emission is merely a release from tension, an anticlimax rather than a climax. The only time I actually get some pleasure from emission itself is when I am making love to a woman who is exciting, who has raised the pitch of my body with a lot of foreplay, visual arousal, or emotional excitement. For women, or for other men, it may be different. It's true that the body is slightly more relaxed after the emission, making the therapeutic work of massage easier. But relaxing the customer or patient is after all the purpose of the massage. Without it a massage has failed in its primary goal, and the customer should be let off without being charged. Indeed in many cases, thanks to bad attitude or sheer incompetence, I have left a massage more stressed and in more pain than I was when I started." Amen, Amen.

Asian and Eastern European masseuses tend to be far more relaxed about emissions, smiling gently and acceptingly at you and shushing away your embarrassed apologies. They are happy to have helped, and they feel compassion for your tense state. They are not looking to add another item to your bill—though some, of course, will try (and I don't blame them for trying if they happen to be poor).

One more thing: Just because I am a man, it doesn't mean I always want stimulation or ejaculation, or that it is men's preferred form of pleasure. Supposing I have an appointment with a sensual and much desired lover immediately after the massage? Unless I am young and bursting with sperm, my performance is endangered by what has happened. My mojo has been stolen, my cup has prematurely runnethed over, and it may even cause a rift with the lover who might say, "What happened to you today? You are always raring to go!" and might not believe my weak explanation: "It was an accident, Honey. The masseuse touched an erogenous zone repeatedly and all of a sudden, I lost control."

Yet, accidents happen, so who are we—or anyone else—to question Divine Intention? The point is that, in the United

States, 98 percent of all my massages had an overwhelming motive: to relieve sore muscles, stress, and an unbalanced body, and because I enjoy massage in its entirety; and not because I wanted sex, which I was able to get from my wife, from three to five times a week, and pretty good sex too, and without charge. So honor this desire of mine, and give me the best massage you can, and let not the thought of sex cross your mind. Do not prejudge me, or even post-judge me. And whether I desire you or not—and as a weak and easily aroused human being, I might briefly desire you—I will honor and worship you for having given me a caring, compassionate, healing, and superb massage. That's all you ask for—or should—right?

Despite the reality that men sometimes don't even *want* a massage to be sexually stimulating, these feelings are not within our control, are they? For we are men—only the highly yogic and self-disciplined among us can exercise perfect control over the pleasure we receive (even the saintly Mahatma Gandhi had to battle sexual feelings until a fairly advanced age). The rest of us can easily be driven bananas by a skilful manipulation of the assigned doses of pleasure—regardless of our power or intelligence in other circumstances. Yes, even the mighty Al Gore was a pitiful sheep at the hands of Molly, if Molly's story about his Portland session with her is to be believed (and if not, she has to be an A Class artist deserving of an Honorary MFA in Fiction to have made up such a long and complicated story). In many such cases, I often think it is *men* who are in need of empowerment.

Now for a story in which I illustrate the above statement. This story takes place in a beautiful country with no name, a country where there is still innocence, grace, and laughter. Here, I once had a massage that, even though I was paying only for a regular massage, was giving me, as a pure bonus from the masseuse, glorious pleasure of the tantric kind. By tantric sex, I mean prolonged sexual play without a goal, without ejaculation. Why? Because the young masseuse, forbidden by the country's rigid social rules from having a boy friend or from premarital sex, seemed to derive great pleasure from arousing me (and possibly other men like me? I wondered later). Though innocent of actual sexual experience—at least she claimed to be a virgin—she seemed to know enough about the male sexual response to take me to the brink, but never to tip me over into ejaculation except perhaps one in twenty times, and almost never once she became good at it.

I will call her Sally. I had chosen her after I noticed she was more giggly and playful than the others and didn't mind my affectionately touching her shoulders and an occasional pat on her bottom. She has the large, almond-shaped eyes and face of an apsara: the kind of apsara whose joy, purpose, and fulfillment proceeds from the love and pleasure they give to men. Her massage of my inner thighs, excruciatingly slow, prolonged the pleasure, the suspense, the anticipation, which is 80 percent psychological. Her fingertips would just graze my balls, and her fingers would tease me by being not in all places, by favoring only a few spots, and therefore waking up a few million neurosensors which were all screaming, like ten thousand African children under a low-flying helicopter throwing out packets of cookies: "Me, me, me! Please, Beautiful Lady, touch me!"

But the big surprise was yet to come. When the massage was nearly over, and she was massaging my chest, I suddenly noticed her thick pony tail of hair, which seemed to rise vertically, then make a hairpin bend and fall down her face or head, sometimes on the left side, sometimes leaning to the right. A woman's hair had always been a turn-on for me. My mother had long, lush hair, and my wife's long, lush hair (after a brief period of cutting it short, she left it long for me, for the remainder of our marriage) was an inseparable part of her sensuousness for me. Now, observing Sally's lush and long ponytail of hair, I reached out for it and touched it gently, put my fingers lovingly around it, and was amazed at its thickness and weight. I began to run my fingers over it, sensuously, almost as if over a tender lover, or as if I had suddenly gone mad and lost control. I held her pony tail and moved it around so as to make her hair fall and graze my chest and neck, caress me even while I caressed it.

Amazingly, she seemed to be excited by this unorthodox use I had found for her hair, and lowered her head to enable me to fully enjoy her hair; she even laid her head on my chest a few times. Yes, on my *oily* chest. That she had thus entered the sensuousness of the moment: that was her gift to me, a totally unexpected gift, thus giving me more and even more of what I had seized, seized at first wordlessly, without asking for permission.

I was like a man who had been lost in a desert for weeks, and was suddenly enjoying the luxury of an unlimited shower in a five-star hotel, or a dip in a gigantic lake. Only, this was a shower of silky hair soothing my chest, my neck, my face, and my eyelids.

From that day onwards, I would look forward to the moment during each massage when I would ask her to unclip her long, glorious hair.

Why? She would invariably ask, almost as if playing with a child: "*Why, why my hair?*" she would continue to ask, even as she unclipped her hair and let its lush fullness drape and tingle my naked body, seeking its crevices and bumps. And then, as she drew her hair up and down the length of my body, especially circling it around my nipples and then, after I had turned over, over my yearning back and my quivering bottom, she kept asking, in the singsong tone of voice she might use with a baby, *Why? Why? Why my hair?* And all the while, she looked like a woman empowered, excited: the thrill she received from witnessing the erotic power of her hair was indescribable. Had I been allowed to check, I could have guaranteed her panties were dripping. For she had discovered Hair Power.

At every massage now, it was *she* who would offer her hair, offer to brush her hair against my nipples, all the while making a babyish noise, as if she was playing with a child. *What hair? You want my hair?! Why? Like this? Ohhh! You like it! Ha* *ha!*shewould say in a singsong voice as she brushed her hair all over my chest and neck, and then, at my request, on my back, buttocks and the back of my legs.

Soon, she became more interested in my balls and in my bottom. She could see, from the view of my legs spread out at a 15-degree angle, that each time she touched my buttocks, anus, perineum, or Balzac, I experienced a little tremor of pleasure and my cock started to grow fatter and longer. Fascinated by her power, she became like a rocket engineer at the Houston Space Center control room, directing the movement of this little rocket of mine, now her personal rocket, her plaything, by virtue of the precise control she had over it, and my helplessness in that prone position, arms stretched, face in a most uncomfortable oval face stand with a hole that could barely accommodate my nose and my eyes.

So it went. Sally had perfected a massage that in its effect fit Oscar Wilde's definition of a cigarette as "the perfect type of pleasure: it is exquisite and leaves one unsatisfied."

One day, her teasing simply did not stop, as I extended the massage from 60 minutes to 90 minutes, and then to 120 minutes. So horny had I become from 1.5 hours of arousal and retreat, arousal and retreat, her tingly fingers etching parabolic curves of ecstasy over my thighs and around the perimeter of my member without once actually touching it, or letting her long, lush hair brush against my nipples, I most of the time closing my eyes to enjoy these rare and beautiful sensations; so horny had I become, that one hour later, when I made love to a certain special and lovely woman only for the second time in six months, I ejaculated within a minute of entering her. Thus, while I did not mind Sally having stimulated me and driven me wild on most other occasions, arousing me almost to the point of madness—it made me feel extremely alive, and alert, every cell of me seemed to be ready to go to war, or to make love if that was an available choice—it proved hugely embarrassing that night, and dismayed my love partner, who, based on our earlier encounter, had expected much better from me.

THE GUANTANAMOING OF PENISES AND NIPPLES

It was in the spectacular island paradise of Samui, in the Gulf of Siam, that all the psychological, social, and legal borders that I had hitherto been aware of, between men and their masseuses, between men's bodies and masseuses' bodies, disappeared for me. Man and masseuse became one flesh; one loving bundle of throbbing, excited flesh, with a number of connection points, including the most intimate one (a naïve visiting alien could easily have mistook this bundle of flesh to be a single creature with eight limbs). But until then, especially in America, the Berlin Wall between subject and masseuse often intrigued, troubled, and vexed me. Or perhaps it was more like the Mexican American border, which at certain points of connection, immigrant-hating Arizona for example, can be quite dangerous and even fatal to the "intruder" in a land that was once colonized by European intruders.

True, thanks to training and licensing requirements for massage therapists in many Western countries, sometimes requiring two years of study, there is far more professionalism and far fewer untrained amateurs offering massages—except for Holistic or New Age types who don't require licenses in a few U.S. states. In easygoing, laxly regulated countries like Thailand and Indonesia on the other hand, almost anyone can start working as a massage therapist without any training; while this is democratic and empowering for these mostly poor people, it carries with it the risk of a few customers being subjected to incompetent or medically risky massages.

But one drawback of some Western masseuses (and I include many countries mentally colonized by the West) is this feeling at the back of their minds: *Oh, I would love to massage the human body; if only half of these bodies didn't come with penises attached to them.* They simply cannot accept the thought that the present model of man, created by an allegedly male God (conveniently created by male prophets), comes pre-fitted with that unholy and horrible thing called a penis, and they punish the poor man for it, making it (and him) shrink and cower and hide in its little dark corner. The maneuvers they make to isolate, quarantine, and neutralize the aforesaid male snake are often so highly creative (and sometimes hilarious) that they merit five low whistles. Many a traditional American masseuse's attitude to a penis is like the traditional American response to terrorists: quarantine them in Guantanamo, where they can be isolated and prevented from attacking the American mainland.

But this artificial division between intimate parts and non-intimate parts is a figment of our compartmentalizing imagination. Which our bodies simply don't recognize, which Nature doesn't recognize, and which is therefore manmade and woman-made bullshit.

On the other hand, many an Oriental woman has no problem with the phenomenon of men having a fleshy appendage between their legs, whether hard or soft. Indeed, it's sometimes the opposite: because you have a penis, you are a blessed, sacred thing. Once, at a New York Korean massage spa in the vicinity of Penn Station, a Korean masseuse who had just (or on a previous occasion) given me a massage passed me in the Men's Locker Room where I was toweling myself dry after a shower. And with a "Hi" and an affectionate smile, she simply touched my penis lightly as she passed. (Lightly patted would also be correct, gently fondled would also describe it— "groped", certainly not.) That was it. It might have been a handshake, but since my penis was out and also available and my hands busy toweling myself, it seemed more proper and respectful to say "Hi!" my more essential and dominant part.

However, imagine if the reverse had happened; imagine if a male therapist had walked through the Women's Locker Room and patted a woman affectionately on her vulva to say "Hi"— the cops would have been there in five minutes, and the poor male therapist marched off to spend the next ten years of his life in a Maximum Insecurity Prison.

I also recall a masseuse I had called in to my hotel in Songkhla, Thailand, and who had appeared anxious and nervous about me when she first entered my room. Within 20 minutes, this mother of three grown daughters had become so comfortable and intimate with me, that, while working on my upper back with her right hand, she rested her left hand on my right buttock for support, her fingers hovering around the entrance to my crack. This is one of the most comforting, trusting, and touching gestures a human being can receive from another being: a gesture which says: *Your body is like my body, I have ceased to feel any difference or separation of identities between us, and I can use parts of you for support without asking for your permission.* It is a beautiful and intimate and warm gesture. Absolutely no fear and trembling about New York State Law or lawsuits alleging violation or sexual harassment.

Far more intimate were my massages with Yu, 27, another Thai masseuse, who in the beautiful little Gulf of Thailand island of Koh Samui became my girlfriend for a while, a part-time girl friend rather, because, though our passion had spilled over into the realm of love (or so I felt) and strong sexual attraction. I would still pay her for the massage (plus a good tip) and she would return to her massage joint, though later she took a week off to live with me in Bangkok. While she was massaging my arm or chest, say, one of my hands would cup her tits, or I might insert a finger inside her pussy and leave it there; nothing like resting your finger in the best and warmest possible spot, the sacred spot, which may indeed heal arthritis and possibly other ailments, vaginal secretions having been scientifically proven to contain hormones that boost immunity and prolong life expectancy. Why not rest one's hand or finger on the bed, you ask? Because that's boring, one is doing it every day. Life is short. You don't have a loving woman in intimate surroundings every day, and this is a gift one can never take for granted—as months and months of post-divorce existence in the New York desert has taught me. (The "scientific proof" that I mentioned two sentences back: may have come in something I read somewhere, though I would not swear that it was in good old *Readers Digest*, which did however surprise and impress me a few years back by publishing an article on why sex is so good for our health.)

The other cool thing about Thai masseuses: Anatomy may be sacred and god-given, and indeed it is, but it is also hilarious at times. So if they find your pecker standing up or staying resolutely sideways over your thigh and thus obstructing the course of Sacred Thai massage justice, they will laugh— sometimes laughing really hard at a dick that seems to be pointing at them or following them around like a pet one-eyed puppy, which these amazing creatures can sometimes end up impersonating. And perhaps a masseuse might tickle or touch it playfully, or make a joking comment. Even if this playful conversation or touching is the limit of how far she intends to go, there's no reason to be a prim stuck-up ass and not laugh along with her. For the nice thing about her laugh (including the laugh of Veronica, my Catholic Catskills masseuse, who was pretty earthy, used the word "stiffy" for erection, and had a low tolerance for bullshit), especially if you laugh along with her, is that it relaxes you: you can see the humor of it, rather than feeling guilty and having to try to explain your erection.

Indeed this particular Thai masseuse, massaging my inner thigh from behind, finds her finger being obstructed by my glans or penile knob, and yet she repeats the move, twice or thrice. She's not going to let a wayward and truant penis obstruct her in the professional duties as a loyal Thai masseuse, is she? And hooray for that! Hooray for the professional dedication of the Thais!

But, to return to the philosophical issue of what is body and what is not-body:

There are those masseuses who in their attempts to avoid, at all costs, contamination by the Big P (pecker, penis, peepee— your choice, take any one from Group A, or take all of me if you wish), arm themselves in a manner calculated to elicit respectful whistles from the designers of the Star Wars Space Shield; their attempts are so heroic they recall the Dutch boy who, to prevent a dyke from flooding his country, plugged a hole with his finger (or his pecker, according to certain subversive alternative historians). But such efforts are doomed, as demonstrated by the philosophical exploration that follows, and which is a tiny bit more sophisticated than "Hey, the love muscle is also a *muscle*, right?! So isn't it your job to release my *muscular* tension?"

Consider: once you begin to break down matter, you first get molecules, and then atoms, and then protons, electrons, neutrons, Bosons, and so on and on (and perhaps even a few morons), and plenty of empty space in between these subatomic particles. And so, despite any optical illusions to the contrary, despite any illusions of separateness, the body is nothing but one big gaping hole or circus tent in which neutrons, protons, electrons are whizzing about like berserk fleas high on amphetamines; head atoms are shooting the breeze with foot atoms, penis atoms are exchanging telephone numbers and friendly hugs with non-penis atoms, and butt atoms are doing it to groin atoms from behind. The borderline between the one and the other, between arms and abdomen, between shoulders and peckers, is a mere optical illusion, a thing of infinite chaos and blindness, which not even the most advanced microscopes can detect.

It would help, therefore, for the sake of everyone's sanity and the sanity of the planet, to think of the entire male body as nothing but the extension of a penis, whose humble and sometimes cunningly disguised slave it is. So the male body is, if you wish, a sub-penis, a proto-penis, a Friend and Slave of the Penis (as in "Friend of the Court") (hey, with friends like these, who needs enemies?). Therefore, your attempt to delude yourself that you are preserving intact your Heavenly Virtue and your Anti-Penile Hymen by not crossing the line between Penis and Not-penis is only a matter of degree, and more a matter of your self-engendered delusion than anything else. A delusion similar to a few fanatic Hindu vegetarians' insistence that *no* one who has *ever* touched meat be allowed to eat in their kitchens or off their plates—or to help in the cooking. (Yes, I know one such dork, an Indian businessman, who lives in a dog-eating East Asian country and putters around town in a minivan built by beef-eating Americans, using a superbly efficient local secretary who is not allowed to enter his kitchen because she is a meat-eater.) But what if the vegetable seller who sold them the vegetables helped himself to a beef kebab while on his snack break, and then, without washing his hands, touched the vegetable that you ended up eating? Similarly, what if the massage customer's hands had touched his Sacred Personal Lingam when having a pee, thus polluting his hand with Sacred Lingam Flakes, molecules, atoms, or subatomic particles? Shouldn't the masseuse, to avoid contamination, also avoid touching her male customers' *hands*?

A final argument: it seems rather arbitrary and fascist to me to so violate the human rights of a particular patch of skin when, after all, we may be nothing more than a congregation of atoms with self-consciousness and an inflated sense of our worth.

And now for a word from and on behalf of Our Nipples. (Clarification: As I have not interviewed enough women to elicit *their* opinions on nipples (all I know is that women's reactions are highly variable, and sometimes even vary within the same day or the same month), the words that follow are spoken only on behalf of the neglected and mute nipples of *man*kind.)

Why are nipples, and sometimes the one-inch area surrounding them, left meticulously untouched by many Western or Western-influenced masseuses, who steer clear of them the way American convoys in Iraq and Afghanistan regard Improvised Explosive Devices?

I imagine the thinking behind it is this: *"But your nipples are erogenous, so they ought not to be massaged. Or else, I would be giving you an erotic massage—which I, being a Pure Moral Being and direct descendant of the Virgin Mary, sure as hell will not."* My counter-question: at what point precisely does sexual excitement begin? How many giddy and tumescent neurons make the quorum that tip a male over into the realm of sexual excitement? I remember the masseuse who, while massaging my chest, made seven to ten broad strokes skirting around and isolating my nipples (which her Podunk or Peoria-situated massage school had probably warned her was Red Alert Area Number Three), and doing so, made me feel weirdly uncomfortable, as if she had arbitrarily divided my skin into two warring zones, untouchable North Korea and friendly South Korea. For in the process, she made my nipples feel touch-hungry, touch-mad, rejected, discriminated against, and deprived of their Human and Nipple rights (even though the Most Honorable Al Gore did not lose control, despite his masseuse's allegations, I could easily have lost control with a masseuse such as Molly, especially if she had nipple-starved me after months of having been so generously treated by Asian masseuses). In any case, how could this masseuse be sure that massaging my neck didn't excite me sexually? Or the backs of my knees? Every spot on my body is potentially erotic, and every soft touch is potentially erotic, the particularities varying from person to person. So the only way to frustrate or completely squash any potential erotic excitement in your subject is either to use sandpaper gloves (and be prepared for a lawsuit or worse), or to abandon the massage profession altogether and to enter a cloistered convent a profession such as that of a religious preacher or of a Republican politician (in which capacity you can engage in sexting and anonymous sexual encounters in public bathrooms until caught). Besides which, what a hateful, ungenerous, perverted attitude to life: to so micromanage it as to scrupulously *avoid* giving pleasure!

Besides, if you massage a person, and he sweats, are you giving him a Sweat Massage? If he feels ticklish, is this because you gave him a Tickling Massage? And if you massage someone's thighs, and he has an erection, or even an ejaculation, how grandiose of you to imagine that you are giving him a sex massage! If a woman were to have an orgasm because I gave her a backrub, even a free backrub, I would exclaim, "Hallelujah! More power to her and her sexuality! She's definitely going to go through her life happy happyhappy!" Because, what does it have to do with me? It's her lucky and blessed body, not mine! Get rid of this omnipotent fallacy of yours that you and you alone are the cause of everything.

A touch of the hands can be erotic; even a conversation, the tone of voice, even when uttering such innocent words as "Is the pressure right for you?" can be erotic. That is part of the vast mystery and fascination of the human animal, our inability to predict and minutely control human responses, including our own. Some women can arouse me by massaging my palms and my forearms, not usually erogenous zones for me or for 95 percent of the human race; I mean, truly, such a woman's touch sometimes pumps vast quantities of blood into the spongy tissue between my legs. And yet, I guarantee even a Ku Klux Klan jury would burst into tears and feel compelled to award me massive damages for a massage during which my forearms were starved of touch.

At other times, the flanks of my upper body are erotic. My nipples are most often erotic, yet there is nothing more frustrating and killing to the massage than my feeling that the masseuse's hands have skirted the nipples, leaving a large area of epidermis around it untouched by human hands, starving for touch! "Discrimination!" my nipples scream, and launch into a brief adaptation of Shylock's speech in *The Merchant of Venice*. "Why leave *us* out? What harm have we done to you? Is it our fault that we are nipples, and not toes? Don't we also need touch, warmth, love, friends?"

To sum up: Eroticism and sex are in the brain. Sometimes, a

female hairdresser giving me a haircut with love, affection, and lack of self-consciousness can make me feel sexy and aroused. I have had an erection while being treated by one of my best dentists ever, a woman dentist at the Bangkok Christian Hospital. Were they giving me sex? Should they therefore stop cutting my hair or treating me? At other times, I have had real intercourse that was so mechanical and depressingly devoid of tenderness or passion that I would have preferred a haircut from the right woman instead.

The lesson: Sex is *all* in the head. To try to control my sexual response is to try to control my mind. Do not try, because you cannot.

THE ZEN OF BALLS AND MASCULINE MAINTENANCE

We've spoken at length in this book about women and penises—a huge subject, one must admit, deserving not just a Chair (or a couch, as Sigmund Freud, the Founder of Penis Envy, might have preferred)—yes, not just a Supreme Court bench, a casting couch, or Chair of Lingam Studies, but an entire university dedicated to research on the subject, and at least a few different versions of *Lingam Monologues* running on Broadway. But how about balls, the humbler and oft-neglected younger brothers of penises?

Speaking of balls or bollocks (as the admirable English with their wicked sense of humor call them), how come there has been no great essay on bollocks, ever? Where is the definitive essay on these jewels of the Family of Man from Ralph Waldo Emerson, Charles Lamb, or Salman Rushdie, who has pontificated on every conceivable subject under the sun? What about the *human* rights of those poor bollocks, their right to existence, information, occasional sunshine and fresh air, and universal suffrage? And why is it that in England, the expression "Bollocks!" is a synonym for "Rubbish!"—a dismissive insult—whereas *dog's bollocks* means the ultimate, the best? Is it possibly because dogs give a lot of quality time to their bollocks, whereas men and women, on the whole, do not?

Well, England may not do its duty, but I, a humble writer, am determined that no convention in the world, no limits to conversational subjects, will stop me. Therefore, consider this chapter to be my humble contribution towards remedying this major lacuna in world literature, and the alternative title of this chapter to be: *An Essay on Bollocks;* or, "In Praise of and Defense of Bollocks."

The good news is that many women and masseuses do have a soft corner for balls—a feeling warmly reciprocated by the balls themselves. Indeed, balls attract women, their magnetism operating on multiple fronts. It's quite charming, this special relationship that some masseuses have with balls: a playful one, which may have something to do with their roundness, their vulnerability, and the pivotal role that balls play in the continuation of the species—they are the fathers of the human race at the same time that they are its babies (in the Thai and Cambodian languages, the word for balls, *kai hum* or *pong khado* respectively, translate literally as "eggs of the penis" or "eggs of the banana"—banana being Thai slang for penis). A win-win scenario.

Besides which, women adore twins, as they adore cute puppies, and it certainly helps that there are two of them, though not often identical. (One-balled Adolf Hitler would have been laughed out of any massage spa outside the Third Reich, and even the most loyal Nazi masseuse would probably have been guilty of quite a few suspicious coughs while she massaged Der Führer's pelvic *Lebensraum*.) So give a woman a chance and no guilt at all, no repercussions, no legal Sword of Damocles, and no kiss-and-tell, and she will play with your balls almost forever, sometimes in indirect ways.

As did the Jakarta masseuse who mischievously rested her bottle of oil on my balls and partly against the edge of my anus. Perhaps because balls don't have the "Forbidden Fruit" or other dangerous connotations that the penis has: while the penis can perform some cute tricks, including sending tiny white missiles into outer space or in the direction of a salivating ovum, it may be a Trojan Horse for vicious viruses, it may jump up and bite you, it sometimes resembles a snake (possibly Rasputin's dick really *was* a snake), and snakes have a reputation for being slimy, tricky, poisonous, and deadly. Besides which, a particular penis may be dirty or unwashed for months, and it could conceivably spray fluids of unknown vintage at you . . . . such unattractive attributes make the dick fraught with many more grave consequences than balls. Also, everyone from your mother to your elder sister has told you to be careful around men's dicks, that they are the source of most of the world's known problems (and a fair portion of the world's yet to be discovered problems). But no mother has warned her daughter against balls, which after all just lie there helplessly, doing nothing at all; they are sitting ducks, so to speak (or duck's eggs, if the Thais were commissioned to enliven the English language). Above all, they are funny!

Now I don't and cannot claim to be—and will fight to the death any imputation that I might be—the world's preeminent authority on balls. I haven't researched them at great length, for one thing, and to be quite honest, I must confess that I haven't studied a single other pair, possibly because I am not a woman, and men's balls bore me to death. The most distasteful part of watching an erotic movie, for me, was that depending on the kinkiness, lack of imagination, or possible homosexual leanings of the director or the cameraman, I might be forced to watch close-up view of other men's balls, and for far too long—time I could have better spent reading *Finnegan's Wake, Gravity's Rainbow,* or *The Music of the Spheres.* I can't speak for my fellow men, many of whom are obsessed with ball games and ball game expressions such as "in the ball park." But, speaking for myself, and only for myself: when a woman gently touches my balls, I am aroused and my penis become erect and starts to leak seminal fluid—perhaps one drop every ninety seconds— which of course, if noticed, might seem like a magical discovery for the masseuses, so they don't stop, it is like they have finally figured out how to operate the safety remote control and, without actually soiling their hands with the Forbidden Dick, have made it dance to their tune.

On the other hand, some women simply don't understand the Zen of balls, let alone of masculine maintenance. As was the case with Pattaya Masseuse "Noo No.8," as she described herself: she simply didn't get it.

You see, ladies—or even if you don't see, and even if you are legally, morally, and politically blinded to this subject, you better understand this—men's balls are a "No Speeding" zone. Just as a neighborhood with a large number of little children will sport "Slow Children" signs on their roads, so too, similar signs, prominent and unambiguous, needs to be placed at about a distance of six inches in every direction from the balls: "Slow, Balls. Maximum Speed: 1 Mph."

But Poor Noo didn't understand. Compassionate, eager, even horny—I say this is vehemently not true of the average Indian or Cambodian woman, but absolutely is of Thailand and Indonesia: that an extremely strong genetic propensity for survival has endowed their women with more than average horniness per capita.

Thus, Thai women make up in lust what they may lack, say, in their aptitude for Quantum Physics or for Existential Theory. So Noo the Horny had of her own accord removed the towel I had draped around my waist (and the fragile "modesty" that it covered) and, as I lay there bollock naked, she had spread my legs from behind while massaging the back of my thighs.

Now that I had turned over, she had my full frontal view spread out before her, and she was probably even more aroused than I. Which is when her hands, like a speeding locomotive on a slippery track, zoomed towards my groin again and again, bringing forth from me a partly self-defensive "Ouch!" especially when these greedy and slippery hands bumped into my balls at way above the speed limit. An instinct for self-preservation had already made me physically transport my member from the side she was working on, forcing it to lean left or right, in the opposite direction regardless of its inherent inclination of the moment. But balls are not so pliable, not so easy to cart around; they don't come with wheels, they are sort of tied down. So here she was, giving me a pretty good massage, but the threat to the family jewels had me up in arms (or should I say, up in legs?). My whole system was on high alert, the Anti-Ballistic Missiles were seconds from launch, because High Command (yes, Their Majesties, My Balls, which ruled my person, being the Reproducing Agents of the Species) had to be saved, and lesser body parts had been authorized to plan and execute suicide missions if necessary.

In any case, many of her strokes, though reluctantly avoiding my balls after I had delivered a firm warning that any further incursions would be repelled with disproportionate and overwhelming force (The Dubya Doctrine), were pushing large quantities of oil deep into my groin. So much so, that, in spite of the shower, which she aided me with, raunchily groping my dick while pretending to help me, and again later when I was changing (whew! I had thought that groping was an exclusively male failing, but obviously I had never been to a Ladies Night at a joint featuring male strippers, or met Noo No.8 before this), I went home and, idly feeling my groin, suddenly had the impression that I had struck oil, and in quantities that made the Persian Gulf seem rather arid.

But the main purpose of this chapter was to give balls their due, their protection, and to speak in Defense of Their Realm. And I hope I have done Their Majesties justice.

What, I haven't done them justice? Okay, let me then give you the story of one more masseuse who had a special affection for balls.

In Phnom Penh, Cambodia, I am in a joint with A-class masseuses and few inhibitions about male anatomy—rare qualities in Cambodia, which suffers from a far milder form of India's moral split personality: social pressure for a public pretence of virtue and sexual conservatism from its women. My usual, experienced masseuse being busy, I nervously try the younger girl, Linda, perhaps 21, who I assume will disappoint, being young, inexperienced, and unacquainted with my peculiar needs and dislikes. But, after I have explained to her that my back, especially my upper back and lower back, needs special attention, she proceeds to give me one of the best lower back massages I have ever had, especially after I have, for a second time, pointed to the inner thighs around six inches below my pelvic fulcrum.

So good is she that sooner rather than later, something is going to happen, now that her hands are now freely roaming from my inner thighs to my balls and up to caress my lower buttocks. All this with the smooth, silky hands of a lovely masseuse who is 22 years old at most. And this dreaded but nevertheless exciting something happens, and when it does, it has this way of spraying into a lower corner of my thigh and the towel to evade discovery. Fearing a discovery in any case, because it may make me feel shy or sheepish, I immediately distract her by asking her to start re-massaging my shoulder. Having diverted her, I mentally assess the damage: so arousing had her touches been that every sperm that was remotely in attendance, and even a few that were legally off on their lunch break, was given the bum's rush and catapulted out within seconds. I am so completely drained it feels as if it could take a long, long time, before my balls will ever feel full again.

There's another reason why masseuses are always more liberal with your rear (which is the preferred access point to the balls) than they are with the corresponding parts in front: because they are getting an eyeful, but without them being caught in the act. Your eyes are not staring them down and their eyes are free to roam anywhere they like without risk of discovery, without having to pretend to be uninterested or casual. Besides, lying face down, you are immobile, unable to suddenly turn around and attack, and in effect harmless—and this harmlessness makes them feel more comfortable and more daring.

More power to them.

Back to Linda: when I turn over, my eyes and hers meet, and she smiles, and this happens around ten times in the next 45 minutes of this two-hour massage, and somehow I notice a greater intimacy in the way we are now looking at each other, it is as if in the episode of the balls, we have shared something intimate, a partial embrace of souls, and she knows it, and feels closer to me.

Pleased at this connection, I return a few days later, and this time she doesn't need a request from me, nor does she ask permission: it is as if her hands are a soft, soft shoe brush, the oil is shoe polish, and she is giving me a gentle but perfect shoe shine—on the back of my balls and buttocks—in preparation for the Grand Inspection by a visiting General or President. How dedicated and unrestrained. Once again, within a few minutes, a few million helpless wrigglers are shot off into the spaces between the interstices of my towel . . . (and shortly thereafter, end their brief, inglorious lives).

Ah, relief. Ah, ecstasy. And gratitude from me, for her kindness. This is why, I keep reminding myself, I should not be so closed-minded. I should be open to trying new masseuses—because sometimes, trying a new masseuse is like trying a new lover. If it turns out nicely, the ecstasy and gratitude of the first time is in a special class of its own, and will always, always be superior to a tenth night with Angelina Jolie or Megan Fox.

Before I end, let me mention another masseuse whose ingenuity was a tribute to women's creativity. She being a mother of two in a conservative country, she was totally in charge; I gave her general directions, but was totally passive on the table. Her technique was to place the towel over my belly and legs in a way that it arced away from her, thus exposing around one-fifth of my pubis and my groin (the side she was working on), the side view of my balls, and the entirety of my inner thigh, but absolutely none of the well-sequestered penis—so that she could never, ever be accused of decadence, neither in this life or the next. And I was grateful for her thoughtfulness, because the pubis and the groin are important, but are often neglected by the prudish. Massaging my thighs starting from above my groin, she made it a point to gently bump against the side of my balls during each up and down motion. I hope her contribution to the universe of Balls is recognized with a honorary PhD from Ball State University (Indiana).

In the hands of an experienced Southeast Asian masseuse, the balls are a major battlefront in the war to subdue men using their superior sexual technique. When the right feathery touch of feminine fingers moves gently over your expectant balls, it can send jolts of electricity throughout your system; it is even better than a woman expertly tonguing your ears and neck, which are also a major turn on for the sensuous man.

IN PRAISE OF PRETENDED
ANATOMICAL INNOCENCE

You would think that an ignorance of anatomy would be a crushing disqualification for a masseuse. In general, your hunch would be correct. But in reality, a partial innocence about the male anatomy (mostly pretended, I realized later—never underestimate the intelligence of women, and don't ever forget that their superior peripheral vision and intuition can leave us men in the dust) can result in lots of good, clean fun, meaningful laughs as well as pleasure for all parties concerned, including for the male being massaged by a woman. It always delights me to notice how often a right-leaning or left-leaning penis manages to sneak up on an anatomically innocent masseuse and take her by surprise, and how despite all her attempts at assuring modesty and propriety, the cunning penis lies in wait and ambushes the lovely hand which, until that moment, had been determined to touch only your boringly legal parts.

The secret is this (and please *do* make a donation towards my Research Fund and Truth Commission if you are a masseuse and obtained this secret from me): As in politics, so in Essential Anatomy: very few men are true centrists. Nearly all of us have penises that lean mainly either to the right or the left. My own dick doesn't even know its own mind: Most often, like my political views, my penis leans to the left; but at other times, inexplicably, it will decide—also like my political views—to lean towards the right. At other times it leans towards the far-right or far-left, rarely even going for a reactionary southwestern inclination, surprising even me, its owner, while on still other occasions, it gets into a playful mood and tries to imitate a low-flying but stationary cruise missile, its shaft hovering at an average altitude of around one inch above my thigh. Why this is so is a mystery I cannot explain, though a probable theory is that it, having a will and an agenda of its own, is trying to hypnotize the masseuse into taking off her clothes and getting into bed with me. You wouldn't expect it of such a tiny fellow, one who doesn't seem to come equipped with any brains, but it/he is a wily seducer, one who outshines me by far.

I have in recent years connected with a woman who has been massaging me quite naked. Meaning, *I* am fully naked; having started formally, with a towel guarding the Crown Jewels, at some point we decided there were no secrets left, that everything I had to show had been seen umpteen times, and to cover myself was sheer laughable hypocrisy and a waste of towels, which, as I was single, I would have to launder myself.

Now this woman, who I shall call Sara, has even pointed out to me after long observation and careful study over the course of perhaps fifty massages with her that my penis follows her in whichever direction she goes while massaging me. And she is really proud of it, it is amusing and flattering to her at the same time—a feather in her cap, if she had a cap. And I must admit she is right most of the time, though the wily little thing foils all predictions, including hers.

In any case, as we are comfortable with each other, most of the time this is a game that helps us pass the time and squeeze a few laughs out of the Unfathomable Absurd, which Albert Camus used up many books and trees, and much valuable time trying to explain. But with the combination of a new and innocent masseuse and a towel or bed sheet, the results can be surprisingly delightful. Because a woman who massages you naked but mechanically is far less erotically arousing than a woman who massages you while you are well-covered, but accidentally touches your penis (and secretly, you have been yearning for that touch of total acceptance, it's been nearly half the point of the massage).

Most Western masseuses will expertly slide the edge of the towel over your penis and around it and then wedge the edge of the towel under your other thigh, thus quarantining your penis and reducing any risk of accidental contact by 98 percent. But this rarely happens with Southeast Asian masseuses, who are more prone to happy accidents (and also, perhaps not so incidentally, to "happy endings."). Perhaps Southeast Asian women, who claim they are used to small and fairly sleepy penises on their usual local massage subjects, have not mentally adjusted to the slightly longer length and excitability of a foreigner's penis. More likely, they are simply *pretending* to be innocent, because they enjoy these accidents as much as the men do—and that it is all a grownup version of the game of hide and seek that can endlessly delight a child, and eternal children like me.

I had another recent experience, going to a massage place when I was down to my last 80 dollars, hadn't been massaged in four days, and desperately needed to save money, despite the massage costing just seven dollars an hour. Not finding my usual reliable, expert masseuse, I reluctantly accepted 21-year-old who said she had had two years of experience. In the massage cubicle, I having stripped and lying face up with a towel covering my privates, she started massaging my left leg. After a bit of that, I was aroused, and told her to move on to the right leg, as my main goal today was to give my hands, shoulders, and back the maximum possible attention. But she delayed moving to the right leg, against which my semi-erect penis was leaning today, camouflaged by the towel. When she got to my right leg, and gradually discovered the contours of my penis by bumping into it from different directions, she just wouldn't stop. She had massaged my left leg for around seven minutes; she stayed on my right leg for around 20 minutes, mostly massaging the thigh around my penis, getting bolder and bolder, and discovering to her delight that her hand could also slip under the penis and massage the strip of skin that was hiding under it. She also learned to move it around, to gently bump into its knob, and to bypass its traffic cop obstructions on her way to my balls. All this time, I said not a word, but simply closed my eyes and enjoyed this totally unexpected gift of pleasure. For I knew that in this country, the penises of foreign men had some sort of mythical reputation, and something within me told me, that she was enjoying herself, that she was fascinated, that for her it was a learning experience and a voyage of discovery; besides which, she was also being kind. Her anatomical ignorance was more than made up for by her openness and an eagerness to learn.

The kindness and affectionate quality of her nature was evident from the way she massaged the rest of my body. When she massaged my arm, for example, she held my hand, as if supporting it, but held it like a lover, with a kind of warmth and affection that I rarely received from a Western masseuse (Lisa and a few like her accepted). Her feeling was communicated in her smile, the personal questions she asked about me and my children and my marriage, and the way her body was so available, pushing against mine even as she continued giving me the massage; my hand was often on her thigh or on her chest, and she let it stay there, almost seeming to signal a welcome, though I didn't take advantage, didn't want to be greedy after having been the beneficiary of so much.

.

RANDOM NOTES ON THE MASSAGE UNIVERSE

While there are many excellent and comprehensive massage books in print, I think they tolerate too much hocus pocus under the umbrella of real therapeutic massage—as if hoping to please everyone and offend no one. Their very politically correct all-inclusiveness makes their judgment suspect and, to the detriment of the profession and its clients, makes massage a field in which anything goes. Also, none of these books expresses a purely consumer or layman's viewpoint, the viewpoint of a receiver, aficionado and major massage consumer like me.

To counter this tendency, this book, while making no claim to being authoritative or comprehensive, energetically expresses its subjective viewpoints, which are enriched by vast experience and are sometimes passionate or tongue-in-cheek.

A few of the following observations apply mainly to Western massage, but the underlying principles are universal.

Yoni Massage for Women's Empowerment.
I am all for it. The website of WhiteLotuseast.com explains yoni massage thus: "Yoni is the Sanskrit word for the vagina that is loosely translated as 'sacred space' or 'Sacred Temple.' In Tantra, the yoni is seen from a perspective of love and respect.

This is particularly important for men to learn."

I say: Amen. Count me in. I am an Eternal Worshipper at the said Temple, and my love and respect for the Yoni is boundless as the Expanding Universe, which by the way is nothing but scientific jargon for the Cosmic Yoni. Not only do I volunteer my services (one free yoni massage a week, my humble and tiny gesture of giving back what women have given to me), I urge inclusion of the Right to Yoni Massage as a sub-clause of the U.N. Charter's Universal Right to Massage.

But are they legal in America? I am not sure, having heard that New Jersey, in a reprise of that old Puritan distrust of pleasure that is always lurking in the American Psyche, recently tried to ban Brazilian waxing. Besides, if they clearly were legal, a franchise called The Great American Pussy Rub would have become the Next Big Thing after Microsoft and Google.

What about the East? Despite the Filipino brouhaha over the rise of lingam massage parlors in Cebu, where the lingam technicians sometimes dressed in schoolgirl uniforms, my Filipino informant, asked whether the poor, oppressed yoni was getting its share, replied, "Not really."

This is a grave injustice, against which women's groups need to march across the planet (Yonis Across America? Yonis Across the Universe?). For let us admit that the massage world, at least in the East, tilts heavily towards lingams—and boy, that is some tilt! If yoni massage were freely and widely offered, women would be more empowered and less easily enslaved; besides which, I am not only against wars fought with guns and bombs, but also regret the endless wars between the sexes, wars that rob humanity of so much of the energy it needs to devote to more crucial causes such as mosquito nets, cheap medicines, and better nutrition for Third World children, and of course, to tackling global warming. Frequent yoni massages would leave us less inclined towards such internecine wars. If the Health Reform Bill placed President Obama in the same history-making bracket as Franklin Roosevelt and Lyndon Johnson, then the launching of the American Yoni Massage Corps to serve the cause of women's empowerment in Third World countries would bracket him along with his other hero, JFK, the founder of the American Peace Corps.

Imagine Shakespeare writing *Hamlet* in 2010. Instead of a speech starting with "Poor Yorick!" it might have begun with: "Poor Yoni!"

Mumbo Jumbo Massages

What I call Mumbo Jumbo massages are massages that are heavy on ritual and mumbo jumbo and short of red meat: meaning, on actual therapeutic satisfaction and relief, which comes from strenuous and conscientious work with the hands. Speaking from vast experience, I say: Beware the Mumbo Jumbo Massage: the so-called "holistic" New Age massages with various names that claim to achieve much of their therapeutic results without touch, but with breathing, words, mantras, laying of warm hands, elbows, stretches, dancing, incense, or whatever. Ritualistic, arcane, pseudo-spiritual, with hints of supernatural effects, this mumbo jumbo becomes a smokescreen, a justification for entitlement. Yeah, do a little mumbo jumbo, and presto, you are a massage therapist, and you deserve fifty dollars an hour, whereas if you were doing a regular job for someone of your caliber, you would be earning eight or ten dollars an hour at McDonalds, twelve dollars tops. How convenient! For me, unless you actually touched me during the entire period of the massage (except when I was turning over), unless you relieved my physical pain and muscle tightness with your kneading and touch for at least 55 of the 60 minutes of the average one-hour massage, you are shirking your duty. And if you want to perform this mumbo jumbo on *your* time, and allow me to decide if it was worth paying for, fine. If not, because of my tight budget, I cannot afford to take the risk of paying you just for mumbo jumbo. Besides, there's something just a bit hokey about a spiritual person presenting a bill: it is a bit like Mother Teresa walking around with invoices, which she slapped onto the foreheads of the dying beggars of Calcutta, even before she picked them up.

Try them *all* if you have an open mind and an adventurous

nature, and have the cash to support them; or "try anything once." I have tried quite a few different massages and therapies, including the Watsu (underwater) massage at Harbin, California, and the Lomi-lomi in Upstate New York. But now, after all these years of experimentation, there is only one kind of massage for me: massage. Which, in my lexicon, means Swedish massage, deep-tissue massage, oil massage, aromatherapy, Esalen, or one their close relatives: hands on, vigorous, engaged, soothing, relaxing, massage that is accepting, nurturing, combining long flowing strokes, kneading, and deep tissue work, releasing blocked energy and irrigating and oxygenating the tissues. Traditional Thai and Shiatsu massages also have their uses, for specific pain relief, but I find them somewhat lower on the soothing and nurturing scale. In top-quality hands, an Ayurvedic (Indian) massage could be outstanding, but I have rarely received one from an intelligent, sensitive, and un-mechanical practitioner, and cannot afford the spas that are priced for billionaires and royalty. Most other massage therapies, in my opinion, are distinguished only by their percentage of bunkum, and while I will tolerate from ten to fifteen percent bunkum during moments of great need and little choice, that is my bunkum limit. Speaking of Reiki—I do not think of it as massage, but as touch retailed to Westerners starved for touch because of a society that is terrified of contact, scared of intimacy and affection, full of rigidly defined boundaries, one that legally punishes contact without full and signed prior permission. For Asians, who are less likely to face such problems—speaking in general, and outside the urban pockets that are beginning to resemble the West and import its neuroses and ills—there is no such need, and Reiki massage must seem quite absurd.

Why Incompetent Massages Can Be Dangerous

And now to speak of bad or incompetent massages, and how they could be positively harmful, anti-social, or worse.

In the ideal massage, the masseuse, at the very least, touches the subject and conveys caring, compassion, and acceptance through that touch. What could be wrong with that?

Except that in real life, there are a few things that could go wrong. The masseuse could be technically competent but feeling stressed or uncomfortable with the client; or else, she could have joined the profession only for the money, while lacking empathy for human beings and their suffering. In such situations, her touch could contaminate the client with her stress, rejection, or callous indifference.

Yet another scenario: the masseuse could be technically incompetent or anatomically ignorant or both, and as a result could strain or damage tense muscles, twist the neck, or awaken dormant problems that she has no talent or inclination to treat; she may even injure a weak spine or break a finger-joint by using too much strength (as the fragility of individuals and their various body parts varies immensely, from pianists, poets, and violinists to football quarterbacks and sumo wrestlers). As a result, the customer could end up walking out of her massage clinic feeling more unbalanced and in more pain than he was when he came in: if he is extremely unlucky, he may even need hospitalization.

I have often been the victim of incompetent massages, especially when I have had to visit an unfamiliar area and was forced to try someone new. On occasion, I was forced to follow a bad massage by desperately hunting for a better second masseuse to heal the imbalance and pain caused by the first one. Some masseuses stubbornly spend too much time on certain parts and then, before they have completed the massage, announce, "Your time is up!" In such cases, a one-hour massage may end with an entire leg or shoulder untouched. I have actually limped out of the office on a few such occasions, feeling unbalanced, with one leg extremely relaxed and stretched while the other, unmassaged leg is extremely tight and in pain. It is the duty of the masseuse to watch the clock so as to ensure a reasonably balanced massage, and also to find out what the customer's special needs are before she starts a massage.

To give a bad or incompetent massage, therefore, is an

irresponsible and anti-humanistic act, because it may actually damage the health of the person who has come in trust in the hope of seeking better health, and has paid for the compassion and healing they were expecting. This is why I think a rating agency ought to randomly and anonymously test the competence of all massage practitioners and award them ratings or even de-license them when there is compelling cause. From a consumer's point of view: if you are stuck with a masseuse whose competence you suspect, ask her to be gentle and to go easy on any thumping or karate chop moves: indeed, not to make sudden moves and stretches without warning you in advance.

Time Matters and Oil Massages

If you are planning to get an oil massage from a new masseuse in a country like Thailand, and what you really need is relief for muscle aches, you better set your time limits and sub-limits well in advance, and signal to her pretty clearly that you're not expecting any oiling assistance in the genitals department—if that's the case. If you don't, you may find her racing through the mundane but crucial parts of the massage, because she has only one thing on her mind: Getting to Your Dick. Yes, getting to your dick and milking it, thus earning the huge tip that she would then be entitled to extort from the sheepish-looking and shrunken post-ejaculation you. Of course you may firmly resist the Big Sister-imposed climax, but by the time you've made this clear nonverbally, with your removing your penis from the scene of action, most of the massage is over, and your back still hurts like crazy.

Advice for the Erotically Inclined

If you are in the mood for a little erotic excitement, and judge the masseuse to be open-minded, ask for a small towel to cover your face while you are face up. Result: the masseuse feels less self-conscious and more adventurous; while you, not knowing what to expect, are likely to feel your senses heightened by the mystery and your desire. Especially if the rest of you is uncovered (though that is not necessary), and you have given permission to the masseuse to massage you in any way she likes. Perhaps, with the addition of a safe word, like "Stop!" or "Stop, and I mean it!" It might be a bit like blindfolded sex.

What to Watch Out for in Asia

You may find, especially in the poorer countries of Asia, women who massage you without washing their hands, or others who have long and dirty fingernails, which could accidentally scratch you and cause an infection. I sometimes carry around a nail clipper, and maybe I should also carry around a tiny piece of soap and ask them to wash their hands before they begin. If there is a language problem, learning the words for yes, no, pain, more, less, stronger, and lighter, might be a good idea, as would having a small diagram of the human body face up and face down, and pointing to the areas where you need more massage.

MASSAGES WE WOULD LIKE TO SEE BUT NOT EXPERIENCE

The Sumo Massage

The Bone Crusher Massage

The Anti-Massage

The Reverse Massage (in which the masseuse lies on the table and you massage her)

The Traditional Swan Maneuver massage (refer to the Kama Sutra)

The Nouveau Swan Maneuver Massage: Which uses a Real Live Swan after the swan has signed a consent form.

The Pair of Tongs Massage (actually delivered with a pair of tongs).

MASSEUSES: GODDESSES AND ASSOCIATE WIVES?

For many years now, especially in monogamously monomaniac, infidelity-despising, and Bill-Clinton-crucifying America, where to have a reasonably intimate connection with a woman other than your wife is not easy, I have looked upon a good masseuse as nothing less than a goddess. And I don't mean this in the banal, woolly-headed, New Age sense of "Every woman has the Goddess in her." For many years now, I have stopped visiting my regular, born-and-brought-up, parentally indoctrinated Church, the Catholic Church. Instead, I now belong to the Church of the Goddess of Massage, at whose temples I worship between two and seven times a week. And each time I receive a blessing, a laying of hands, from one of the better goddesses, like Lisa—soft, accepting, loving, healing, nurturing, enlivening, empowering and sanctifying—I am healed, and can face the world with lightness, a smile, a feeling of relaxation, and an assurance that life is after all worth living. Or at least until the next massage.

To some men, a good masseuse may approach the status of a goddess, a mistress, a caretaker, and even a wife. For many years, I denied that there was a sexual or romantic element in my massages. To be fair, my wife was mostly tolerant and broadminded, not just receiving massages herself—brief ten-minute ones from me, and regular ones from professionals—

but also occasionally presenting me a massage gift certificate for Christmas or for my birthday, sometimes recommending a particular masseuse by name. However, like one of my later girl friends, she would sometimes seem jealous, which would make me respond defensively. But now that I have much greater respect for women's remarkable intuition, I realize my ex-wife's jealousy wasn't entirely misplaced, even though I was a lot more self-disciplined and less wild than in my unchained post-marital days (like when my possessive Javanese girl friend lay in bed next to mine and watched clueless as the Balinese masseuse, perhaps aroused by inter-island rivalry as well as a little lust, slyly reached under the towel to probe my hot zones). Because massage is a form of marriage, and I may be a natural polygamist, genetically designed for polygamy-friendly ages and cultures rather than this repressive and humorless monogamous age.

Is massage a form of marriage? Well, try looking up the usual American yellow page directories (which I was often forced to do in the Pre-Google era in many a strange city, when desperately in search of a massage). Is it not curious that the "Massage" listing is sandwiched between "Marriage Counselors" and "Mattresses"? The symbolism that I perceive: when you don't spend enough of your married life doing fun things on a mattress with your spouse, you might end up finding someone else to do fun things on a mattress with. And if you don't (and even if you do find that partner to have fun with), you may then have to consult a marriage counselor, while also getting massages to knead out your marital pains, your frustrations, and your epidermal hunger.

Thus it has often occurred to me that like geishas, who acted as intimate companions, entertainers, and lovers to Japanese men whose wives had stopped giving them the playful and romantic partnership they once did—masseuses may to some extent supplement wives and even perform a healing, supporting role that permits men to remain sane and prevents families from breaking up. But as women have sexual needs too, which their husbands may not fully satisfy (they might not be billionaires, for example, or too prone to sadomasochistic practices), they too often need masseuses or masseurs. (Whether or not these masseuses or masseurs become associate husbands, I leave a woman theorist with the appropriate Harvard, Brown, Berkeley or Princeton advanced degree to decide.) For there are bound to be women who feel that their husbands don't touch them enough, don't pay enough attention to all parts of their bodies, and who go for the main thing—that sacred and magical area between a woman's thighs—too quickly and come too soon—after which, according to many standup comediennes, they instantly turn over and start snoring. Such women's bodies may suffer from a deep hunger that needs more meticulous and loving care—which, in the absence of a Kama-Sutra-savvy lover, may need to be provided by a masseuse or a masseur.

In any case, I have no doubt that sexual frustration and bad marriages (or periodically stormy marriages like mine), which like death and taxes will always be with us, are part of the reason why people need massages. To pretend that the two are totally unrelated is so unrealistic that a masseuse who thinks thus deserves to be debarred from the profession for being so clueless about her subjects and about human psychology.

If you doubt the comparison of massage to marriage, take this test: How many of you have been touched by your spouses, gently, unhurriedly, and erotically on your: underarms, flanks, back of knees, behind the ears, toes, on the crease between the buttock and the thigh, and every square inch, crease, and fold of your pelvic region, especially those hidden creases nestling between your thighs? Ninety percent of men are touched on fewer parts of their bodies by their wives than they are by their massage therapists (and to be fair to wives, many of them have jobs and lead far too stressful lives to give their and their husbands' bodies their just due, thus requiring specialist intervention; though, having glanced through a few recent issues of *Cosmopolitan* Magazine, I suspect few of men's secret spots remain secret any longer). Indeed, a spectacularly talented masseuse can arouse and awaken erogenous zones or parts of you whose existence your wife never knew of, which even you didn't know of, which in fact didn't exist until your masseuse brought them into existence, like the Almighty God sending up a fresh island from the bottom of the ocean. And once awakened, you are left yearning and completely at her mercy for the next few massages. Indeed, on more than one occasion, a masseuse has pointed out to me a bump or cut or some other damage to my body that I was unaware of, perhaps in the nick of time before it grew into a malignant tumor or a more serious problem.

Oh sure, I had real pains all the time—98 percent of the time, except when returning for a quick second or third massage from a beautiful masseuse I had become enchanted with in my later, lonelier, less-loved years. Tightness in my shoulders and arms from bending for long hours over a laptop, fibromyalgia, Myofascial pain, Chronic Fatigue Syndrome, pains in my feet, thighs, and buttocks, some owing to flat feet and a podiatric racket in which rock-hard inserts would be prescribed as a corrective, inserts whose steepness and hardness caused pain to radiate all through my body—the cure being far worse than the disease. I tried regular physical therapy, which mildly strengthened my back, but was no substitute for massage, just as a pop melody or a jingle is no substitute for a Mozart symphony. But which came first: the body aches or the marital pain, the feeling of being insufficiently loved, cared for, worshipped, and touched? A question not easily answered, but worth researching with Kinsey-like integrity and labor, unless we're simply aching for quick, convenient, and moralistic answers to match our prejudices. Besides, in the first fifteen years of my marriage I was blessed with a far greater libido than could be satisfied in my three to five weekly lovemaking sessions with my wife; some of that excess sexual energy could have surfaced as a yearning for massages, during which I could be legally touched by women other than my wife.

So massage is an unrecognized form of marriage, except that in massage, polygamy and polyandry are tolerated and often encouraged, and homosexual marriages are as legal as heterosexual ones. Or else, there are monogamous interludes sandwiched between occasional affairs, and sometimes, a promiscuous run of one-afternoon stands. You may use a separate masseuse every day of your life, or have two or three masseuses work on your body simultaneously—and no one except perhaps the Pope or your Victorian spinster aunt is gonna look at it as anything but a therapeutic quest at best, and as delicious and wholesome fun at worst, as harmless an eccentricity as eating your Big Mac in a different McDonalds each day of your life. Because a large number of the planet's residents, emerging from a Darker or more Repressive Age, have entered a more permissive, sensual, and liberated age. This book is meant to celebrate this happy development and furnish you with ideas on how to fulfill and spice your dreams—and that of your lover, wife, or husband . . . and of their lovers and masseuses.

WHEN MEN MASSAGE MEN

Scene: Miami Beach, 1999. The long strip of beach, residences, motels, hotels, and restaurants starting from above South Beach, running up through middle-class and posh neighborhoods like Bal Harbor, and then past the nudist Haulover Beach and to the Sunny Isles section in the 170s, lined with endless condos, hotels, and motels, was my variable home for the first three months of 1999. I was here fleeing domestic disharmony and trying to finish a book-in-progress, and for a month, I lived in a middlebrow motel room with a view of the beach. And sometimes, I needed to call in a male massage therapist because the women seemed to be busier and more expensive (the legendary James Brown notwithstanding, the massage world is *not* a man's world).

On one such day, when the masseuses seem to be either busy or hiding behind their answering machines, I call a guy named Jay, who cannot come (no pun or offence meant, but I do have this slight apprehension that a male massage therapist might be gay and, in the privacy of my room, lose self-control and . . .). I mean, Jay is too busy to come, so he puts me on to his Staff Sergeant (just kidding!), Mike, who arrives at my door soon thereafter.

In the Miami *New Times,* men seem to go for a song: a 1.25 hour massage from Robert Allen, therapist to the Atlanta

Olympic Games: $40. Imagine that! For forty bucks, you wouldn't even get a blind, one-armed masseuse in America! (Speaking of blind masseuses, I remember running all the way around Chiang Mai in Thailand searching for the blind masseuse joint, for it gave me such a kick to imagine the masseuse accidentally stumbling onto my third leg or the misplaced cucumber . . . "Oops, so sorry!" "No problem, help yourself! And while you're at it, why not have a ball?") Whereas women command such high fees because they are favored both by men (the pigs!) and also by other women, feminists especially (oh, the piggies!)

Mike's fee is $35 for the hour, and he arrives at your door, which means you don't have to drive through stop-and-start Miami Beach traffic, a mishmash of senior citizens and drug dealers, and find a parking spot—a steal of a deal, and sensible, because of my strained finances. With Puerto Rican or Cuban looks, this medium-built man has a slightly pudgy face and mildly wavy hair. Though I am apprehensive and defensive, evading his eyes and keeping my towel firmly in place over my member to forestall any misplaced conclusions or stumbles, he ends up giving me a fairly proficient massage. He ends by saying, "It was a *pleasure* to massage you." And I think: "I hope you don't really mean it. Or else, I will be forced to fire you. Or at the very least, to charge you for your pleasure."

I called him again, two days later. Besides being a lot cheaper than women—now, please leave that thought as is, and don't try to take it any further—he was a no-hassle guy, always available, grateful, appearing at your door within 1.5 hours of your phoning him.

Anyway, I decided to be a bit more free-tongued today, to be an investigative journalist. How did he deal with his female massage subjects and their bodies? I asked. "Some of them *insist* on *not* being covered. Then I just ask to turn down the lights." Strange, that he himself preferred not to look at these women who wanted to air their assets; in his place, I might have asked, "Can I turn on *all* the lights? Please? And bring my camera along the next time?" (No, just kidding.) And though I didn't ask if he was gay, I decided to bring matters a little out into the open—figuratively speaking, of course (I thought talking about it might solve the problem—the Sigmund Freud fallacy that I still hadn't completely abandoned at the time) by saying, "I am embarrassed that I sometimes get erections during a massage." He said half the men he massaged got erections. Hearing this, I felt mightily relieved and a little relaxed, for a while. Even my dick took a mini-break.

But as he is massaging my chest, he avoids touching my nipples and I, burning with nipple neglect, speaketh thus: "Hey, Bud, what about them poor little buds?!" No, joking, I actually say something more cunning such as, "Could you go crosswise from the shoulders downwards?" demonstrating with a flat hand moving over my chest *without* careening James Bond-like around the perimeter of the Danger Point, the Little Hill on the Fool, I mean my La Nippolio. Coz hey, man, the perimeter is a mental perimeter, and life is short; so fuck perimeters, parking meters, and talking meters.

So he does, and he does a good and nearly sexy and soothing chest and stomach massage, his hands stroking the sides of my trunk and reaching slightly under my trunk.

At which point, the trouble starts. For it didn't matter, male or female: in those days, I would still get an erection when touched in certain highly erogenous zones like the thighs, buttocks, nipples, or lower abdomen, and sometimes the flanks of my trunk (though, unlike a man, a woman with soft hands could touch even my hands and give me a hardon—sometimes even the mere expectation of a woman touching me might give me a hardon). The erection embarrasses me, but I somehow deal with it, because a massage is like medical treatment: the relief of pain is the foremost goal, and you are not going to stop yourself from going to doctors just because they make you wear those silly open-butt gowns and perform painful prostate examinations, are you? But still, I am terrified of an accidental ejaculation, and wish to ask him how other straight men handle such situations. But I don't.

Once again, when he starts to massage my infamous right

leg, and his touch includes my penis, though sideways and "accidental", it causes my peepee to metamorphose again into something greater than itself. And later, when he lifts both of my legs trying to bring my feet and knees up in a stretch towards my chest, a full erection rises like a flagpole. The erection and the leg stretch conspire together to dislodge the towel, which falls off my body, and I don't replace it, leaving my cock standing just like that (I silently lecture myself that I must overcome this "embarrassment" about natural things like my body and bodily phenomena, having just talked to him about this, and besides, I am mildly curious to see what might happen; even though I wouldn't be cool enough to handle a joking, "Oh, so you *are* rather glad to see me, are you?").

I now realize the stiffy must have been a provocation, if he was indeed gay. For, having made forays towards my pubic boundary while massaging my stomach, he suddenly brushes my penis with his hand as if casually and accidentally, and when I do not object to that initial movement, if indeed it was accidental, he goes on to start a single, unequivocal stroke. At which point, even before the conclusion of his first downward stroke, with split-second speed, I stop him with, "I am not looking for that!" Later, I am embarrassed and angry with myself (and him), thinking, *God, how could I have allowed myself to get into such a situation?*

So that was as far as things went with my male massage therapists in America. Though a few undercover emissions, because when lying face down, one cannot react quickly enough to stop a stroke that is too arousing. And while touch is not always gender-neutral—sex being nearly all in the mind—it sometimes is, especially if the male therapist has soft hands.

Luckily, the incident with Mike happened late in my American experience, and in a hotel room—hotel rooms are notorious for inspiring impure thoughts, can't blame anyone; a good friend of mine used to assert that if you placed a healthy man and woman together in a room, and both were sure that no one else would ever find out, they would sooner or later end up fucking. Regardless of the truth of his theory, the potential for such embarrassing situations partly explains why, for sixteen years in America, even in health clubs like Jack La Lanne, I always preferred a masseuse to a masseur—when available. Blame my genes and upbringing, if you like: but barring a real handshake, a hand on the shoulder, a hug from a close friend, and one awesome masseur at the Bally's Hotel in Atlantic City, I am not fully relaxed about a man touching my body (nor would I bend to pick up a fallen piece of soap in a Greek bathhouse). And a massage is one place where I want to be feel relaxed enough that it would be okay, even nice, if I drifted off to sleep while it was in progress. Is this too much to ask for— to feel comfortable during a massage I am paying through my nose for? But even when forced to choose a masseur, I would try to avoid he-man types who treated their male subjects' bodies roughly, as if fearful that some tenderness or softness might signal homosexuality—which would destroy their reputation and their self-image. I preferred those with softer hands, and those without macho affectations. Because in addition to pain relief, part of what I look for in a massage is softness, tenderness, and mothering. And men, whatever else they may be superb at, including algebra and genocide, are not their best in these latter areas.

On the other hand, as I do passionately believe in equal rights for men: I know from a few online forums that whenever a male massage therapist suggests he is not getting enough business simply because he's male, he's shouted down by colleagues who dislike the truth when it doesn't suit them or fit the current politically correct platitudes. I do hope more and more men get well-paying jobs giving massages—not just to the men who prefer men, but jobs giving sensual massages to needy women starving for the touch of male hands on their bodies, and perhaps even their secret parts. (I have in the past fantasized that I could do a pretty decent job of giving a woman a sensual massage, but I also suspect it is a lot harder work than it seems, being about 20 percent inspiration and 80 percent perspiration.)

SUMMING UP: WHY MASSAGE IS BOOMING

As I write this final chapter, I realize that the law of diminishing returns applies to massages as well as to love affairs and ice creams—when you have had 3,500 of anything, you probably won't be as ecstatic about the 3501st one as you were for the first and the hundredth. But my enthusiasm in principle for excellent, humanistic massages, and their importance to mankind, has not diminished.

To sum up: I am all for clarity, honesty, and a lack of hypocrisy, and for the right of both the masseuse and the customer to choose the massage he or she wants to be part of, without coercion or Big Brotherly restrictions, and provided the giver of a non-sexual massage is technically proficient and does not make the customer feel like a criminal just because he happens to be a male. One way to reduce the possibility of embarrassment for women therapists is to have properly advertised and legalized sensual massages (by therapists who have *freely chosen* to practice this form) widely available everywhere, so that men will not go where they are unwelcome (just as smokers do not willingly choose hotels where smoking is prohibited). It would also help if the former group clearly advertised their services as non-sexual; and, if they so preferred, to confine their practices to other women.

But following years of experience, reflection, and initial denial on my own part, I now believe that but for the abundance of sexual starvation, and but for men not getting enough sex, and perhaps almost equally often, women not getting enough sex (and the sex of their fantasies besides), the demand for massages would plummet to perhaps one-fourth of their present number—and that the demand crash would result in far cheaper regular massages. After all, many licensed massage therapists, even those studying the subject for a year and a half (and many have done much shorter courses), have less than half the education of an average registered nurse, who starts at around $20 an hour in the U.S. It is the sexual and intimate quality of massage and its feeding of the human hunger for nurturing touch, that gives massage a premium far beyond its labor value. (And of course, I believe that outstanding masseuses deserve to be paid in proportion to their excellence.)

However, such an ideal society is still far from realization, and sexual starvation at least to a mild degree is probably going to continue for a long, long time, in most of the world, and to a much greater degree in the repressed countries. Meanwhile, as the inhibitions and hypocrisy surrounding massage gradually diminish, my guess is that massage establishments will continue to boom and prices will not fall significantly anytime soon.

You could say I am a dreamer (and yes, that John Lennon song and the Beatles in general have influenced my thinking in a major way). But allow me, please, to give voice to my dream: that we return to a more intimate form of society, one in which massages are exchanged, bartered, or donated free in volunteer service, in temples of skin-love, much the same way that once upon a time, in ancient Rome, and even in India, I believe, temple courtesans freely gave their bodies to devotees in honor of the god or goddess they served. (For in the end, as the final Beatles song goes, *the love you take is equal to the love you make.*)

Note that it is not only men who derive sexual pleasure from massages. I once met a lesbian who massages only women, even though she doesn't hate men—because she's getting paid for her pleasure, besides doubling her chance for a Saturday night date.

Meanwhile, until the problem of global sexual famine, which affects billions (though some of them might be unaware of it, or unwilling to admit it), and which underlies much war, aggression, hatred, cheating, and genocide, is solved, it is cruel and even dangerous for authorities to stop, curtail, or harass the relatively mild and benevolent relative of sex that is massage in its various forms—even when it has a clearly stated sexual component. Such suppression and harassment still takes place in many parts of the world.

On the other hand, in countries without legal hurdles to massage, there has been an increasing tendency to over-commercialize, the worst examples of which I consider to be expensive and yuppie-serving spas and The Great American Body Rub franchises, where the menu includes items such as just neck and shoulders, or just back, as if the rest of the body were some pariah. All of which seems to corrupt the original spirit of it (when will they start offering massage just for the middle finger or the right ear lobe? I wonder). To capitalistically exploit massage (as takeover specialists buy up mammoth corporations, chop them up into tiny parts, and sell these parts for a big profit) is no better than to sell sex or to sell water or to sell love—things which, in an ideal world, should never be sold.

The over-commercialization of massage has attracted many of the wrong type of people into the profession, including some who actually have no love or empathy for their fellow human beings, but who see it more as a quick money-milking (or customer-milking) business than as a vocation or a mission. I find a few Chinese massage establishments in New York to be particularly guilty of this extortionate attitude, and my hunch is that this happens because the owners exploit their employees, pocketing the entire fee upfront. And the workers, because of their ignorance or perhaps illegal-visa-status, are forced to work just for tips, which they must fight for or extract using dubious methods.

But it also happens elsewhere. In 1999, in a beautiful resort north of San Francisco, the masseuse confessed to me that her share of the $80 massage fee was just $25. This is unconscionable: it should be illegal for any establishment to pocket more than 30% of a massage therapist's fee, no matter what its excuse.

Meanwhile, as the West has become more prosperous and more liberal in theory, more and more people there and in the dizzily developing and rat-racing sections of the developing world, infected by the globalization bug, lead lives of lonely, neurotic, and touch-less desperation (as powerfully depicted in *Atomised* or *Elementary Particles,* the novel by French author Michel Houllebecq).

Therefore, massage ought to be encouraged and subsidized as a humanistic, philanthropic activity (are you listening, Bill Gates?), and as a legitimate branch of medical and psychiatric treatment. It could reduce crime and alienation, besides being an antidote to depression and stress, two of the major scourges of contemporary civilization. America and certain other parts of the world periodically experience a laudable swelling of the altruistic impulse, which results in such episodes or movements as The Sixties, the Peace Corps, Hands Across America, John Lennon's *Imagine,* or "Have You Hugged Someone Today?" How about a People's Massage Movement, in which people volunteer to massage others for no money, but simply as an act of goodwill and their simple and concrete personal contribution to world peace? With the slogan: *Touch Someone to say I Love You?* How about a Massage Corps in line with the Peace Corps? There's no reason, at least in that future, ideal world of John Lennon's "Imagine," for any human being to be starved of touch. (In Cambodia, the traditional massage can cost as little as 6000 riel or $1.50 for an hour, or slightly more than a very basic meal, and at that price is truly a widely affordable people's massage.)

The Beatles, and John Lennon, got it almost right. "All You Need Is Love" might be an exaggeration, but it is not far from the truth. A truth that we need to assert and practice far more frequently so that it might counter the increasing influence of another fairly well-known saying: No Money, No Honey.

Book III
LINGAM AND YONI MASSAGE
A Safe Sex, Anti-War,
and Economic Recovery Tool

[To be read with a bucket of salt and three large scoops of irony]

To think that, like Buddhism, lingam massage was invented in India, but that you are far more likely to hear of it outside India? For I was completely unaware of it until I accidentally stumbled upon the expanding Great Filipino Lingam Massage Debate.

That was when I discovered that professional lingam massage was something of an enviable and exclusive specialty, like cardiology, angioplasty, neurosurgery, or rocket science. Not only was it an esoteric art practiced by a few professionals (known in private circles as The Priestesses of the Holy Rod), its very existence, like that of tantra (of which it is a part), was known only to a few connoisseurs.

First, to clear the air and explain what a lingam massage is *not*: it is *not* a dickie massage. Neither is it some variant of abusing the wicked stick, adjusting the antenna, beating the pud, burping the baby, choking the chicken, couch hockey for one, cranking the love pump, debugging the hard drive, greasing the three-legged cow, jerking the gherkin, or Lubricating the Love Monkey. Or shaking your banana.

It's not the traditional Happy Ending either (and I'm not talking about Hollywood movies or Harlequin Romances), though it may lead to a mind-bogglingly spiritual and transcendent happy ending.

So what *is* a "professional lingam massage"—the kind that had the powerful Philippines Roman Catholic Church, led by it pink-capped generals, training its heavy artillery at some delicate and vulnerable Filipina belles? (The Philippines, a country comprised of thousands of islands and spectacular beaches, is also a country of great contradictions, with some of the hottest, sexiest women, who are outstanding kissers like Indonesian women--and along with this, the ubiquitous presence of Catholicism and widespread opposition to legalized abortion.)

My undercover investigation revealed that while the West expends its fabled ingenuity in developing Star Wars defense systems, genetically modified eggplants, and more scrumptious pigs, it is the East, in places like Singapore, Malaysia, and the Philippines, that concentrates on perfecting the art of living: for example, the gracious, noble, and vital art and science of Lingam Massage (whose secrets, I now believe, ought to be deposited in a time capsule and buried in a deep underground phallus-shaped vault for the benefit and happiness of future generations).

Thanks to the Internet, the YouTube, and jet aircraft, however, lingam massage may soon be as much a piece of our common planetary heritage as tea bags, Big Macs, and Spiderman.

The website of Article Doctor explains: "The Tantra lingam massage is a *spiritual* tradition, which had its origin in India . . . about 4,000 years ago. Hence tantra can also be stated as a form of yoga." Yoga to discipline the notoriously unruly male member, also known in various circles as the the baby basher and the heat-seeking moisture missile? Now that makes sense—it's a no-boner! Though 20 years of solitary yogic meditation in the midst of the Sahara Desert on a diet of boiled brown rice and water blended with stale tofu might be a more effective strategy for taming the one-eyed monkey.

The website of White Lotus East is somewhat more explicit: "The goal is to massage the Lingam, also including testicles, perineum and Sacred Spot (prostate) externally, allowing the man to surrender to a form of pleasure he may not be accustomed to."

Right, baby, count me in: around five years of daily practice should help me to get accustomed to this kind of pleasure.

And on YouTube, Carolena explains: "It's about the *journey* . . ." (meaning orgasm is not the goal), adding that lingam massage can heal trauma and "awaken your man's Inner Clitoris."

Next stop: your man's Inner G-Spot. Followed by his Inner Vagina and his Inner Uterus.

As a man who had recently experienced a world of trauma and whose Inner Clitoris needed a healing jolt of greased lightning, I decided to investigate.

My informant, a fantasy novelist from the Philippines resort island of Cebu, where lingam massage was the explosive issue of early 2010, trumping global warming and Tiger Woods's multiple mistress scandal, tells me his Inner Clitoris is throbbingly awake thanks to having visited two local lingam massage joints named Authentic Lingam Massage and Chuva-Chuva. In Chuva-Chuva, he says, the masseuses dress like schoolgirls, and both joints offer "a one-hour whole body massage plus lingam, all in for P900." Wow, that's less than the *tip* you'd have to pay for a plain old "happy ending" in New York! It's what you might have to pay simply to take off your shirt at one of those forbidding Great American Shirted Back Rub joints.

Further, added my excited informant, "in a hand job, they simply oil the organ and masturbate it. [Ugh!] The lingam massage is more elaborate as it includes the thighs, testicles, and other parts before the doing the conclusive masturbation."In other words, more bang-bang-bang for your buck.

Why do men climb mountains? Every school child knows that ("Because they are there."). Why do men need lingam massages? According to the website of White Lotus East, "to learn to relax and to receive," and to "experience their softer, more receptive side"—unlike their usual, goal oriented mode.

Whereas the website of the Filipino "Lingam Massage Venture" (displaying a photograph of a bevy of sultry beauties whom I would any day trust my lingam with), ventures further: "Men, being competitive usually suffer from anxieties and frustrations. It is believed that men keep a lot of their stress in the abdomen and pelvic area."

True, that's where I keep most of mine (except for the tiny bit that I hide inside my socks for emergencies); but glad to have official, independent confirmation from an authoritative source. The site goes on to explain that its lingam specialists (all women—what a delightful coincidence) were trained by a tantric priest based in Malaysia and Singapore. (Sadly, India, birthplace of tantra, is no place to hunt for a good lingam massage; you might get arrested merely for having made the mistake of *asking* for one. But, had it been otherwise, the Chief Tantric Priest of the Lingam Massage Division might have been titled Swami Lingacharya of Dickenballapuram Mutt.)

The Anti-War Consequences of Focused Pleasure

Returning to the delightful subject of Inner Clitorises: Now I truly believe if only many a world leader's Inner Clitoris—which is often in a coma—were to be kicked awake by some lingam massage experts, millions of lives could be saved by avoiding needless war.

If you are anti-war, you've no option but to be pro-lingam massage, the ultimate anti-war weapon. (Imagine t-shirts that proclaim "Peaceniks for Lingam" and "Hell, No, We Won't Go . . . Without Lingam!"). Frequent lingam massages (which, as one website claims, "allows the man to experience his softer, more receptive side and experience pleasure from a non-traditional perspective."), might have made of many a warlord a softer, gentler man who would not have recklessly dragged his nation into unjust, useless, and unwinnable wars that destroy countries and people. For it has been repeatedly observed that men's fascination with guns, missiles, and large, powerful gas-guzzling cars is a direct consequence of their quest for phallic substitutes to overcome their sexual frustration or their feelings of sexual inadequacy. (You know what I mean: the old male obsession with size matters.)

Therefore, I strongly suggest amending every national Constitution to require that Presidents and Secretaries of Defense undergo lingam or yoni massages twice every week in the interests of world peace. Lest I be accused of anti-yoni-ist prejudice, I also suggest that men be compulsorily taught yoni massage in high school, so that when the legislatures and seats of government increasingly fill up with women, and when women become warlike (well, that's what the experts now claim—that violence is an inevitable and gender-neutral outcome of power), men can pacify them with yoni massages.

Behind the Philippines' explosive lingam massage debate—as polarizing an issue as health care reform in the U.S.—lies the country's dual colonial history and mixed cultural ancestry: liberal relaxed Southeast Asian island culture and genes warring against the colonial legacy of a morally uptight Catholic religion and hellfire blah-blah, resulting in a split personality.

The crux of the debate: Does lingam massage promote health, and if so (or if not), is it immoral? Do we *have* to choose between Spa Heaven and God's Heaven, or could we perhaps visit them on alternate evenings?

Even Cebu's Cardinal Vidal, joining calls to investigate spas offering "indecent" services to their clients, declared: "Because if it promotes immorality, they should be stopped."

But how can a *spiritual* practice promote immorality? And why is the Cardinal taking such a hard stand against a therapeutic procedure that could avert prostate cancer? Why is he angry with those lovely prostate milkers, milkmaids doubling as Florence Nightingales? Still, city councilors, possibly prodded by the Cardinal's displeasure, asked the Cebu City Anti-Indecency Board to investigate if "lingam massage" joints are involved in "indecent and lewd practices."

However, in the same organ (Cebu Daily News), columnist Ricky Poca accuses men of using lingam massage for one thing only. I quote:

> The advertisement says lingam massage is good for the prevention of prostate cancer but many of its customers are young men. It's a hit . . . because it provides tremendous pleasure for men without having to engage in sexual intercourse.
>
> Personally I think it should be [investigated]. What lingam offers is simply sexual pleasure, although I know that some men welcome it. For them, they are engaging in safe sex, not necessarily therapy against prostate cancer.

Should massage be investigated because it gives pleasure? If so, why not also investigate beer, music, and sunsets, all of which also give pleasure? Nevertheless, I hail his column's positive implications: that lingam massage is a stone that nails two birds: prostate cancer as well as STDs and AIDS! Indeed, an NGO's or philanthropist's wet dream!

Admittedly, the lingam massage trend could upset many women—girl friends, wives, and perhaps just lonely women looking for a warm tumble in the hay—who are now left to fend for themselves by men whose Inner Clitoris is in Seventh Heaven. But so long as it is in the interests of safe sex, one of the Holy Icons of the modern age, why object to it? Well, of course they are going to object to any procedure in which they get left out; so why not also offer free or discount yoni massages to the women who are complaining?

Besides, one happy benefit of lingam massage is safe sex, Bill Gates's AIDS-fighting billions could perhaps be put to better use in starting Universities of Lingam Massage, and to finance lingam startups—perhaps to the tune of the Rolling Stones song "Start Me Up."

Meanwhile, at the website of sunstar.com.ph, the lingam advocate Lorenzo Ninal fumes at Filipino Puritanism:

> Because ours is a culture that finds certain innocent words referring to some parts of our anatomy "obscene."
>
> The words I am referring to are penis, genitals, orgasm, ejaculation, masturbation, and other terms that *you, with your puritan upbringing, wish did not exist at all.* [Emphasis mine]

But they exist, after all, these wondrously neat gifts of God to humankind, so one might as well grow up, right?

Meanwhile, Cebu's police chief, under attack from the Puritans, explained that "the police have to catch a masseuse in the act of doing something indecent before they can take action." (I would gladly join the police force if assigned to this job, and promise not to accept kickbacks—well, at least not in cash.)

While in the *Cebu Daily News*, Honey Yoo, owner of Authentic Lingam Massage, defended her service as a widely accepted "wellness" massage. "It is accepted in strict Singapore and widely embraced in Muslim Malaysia, practiced in Egypt, Thailand, New York, California and London," Yoo said. Fair enough: what's good enough for Singaporeans and New Yorkers is good enough for us.

But Yoo goes further and uses globalization and competitiveness to make her pro-lingam case, urging openness to new ideas and asking, 'How will we become globally competitive if we will immediately judge and mislead our customers?'

Why not go even further? I suggest that lingam massage be used not just as a tool for safe sex, world peace, and the prevention of prostate cancer, but also for a global economic recovery. In just the last 4 years, the world has lost around $5 trillion to $10 trillion to pointless wars, dangerous and fantastically expensive weapons systems (male toys), and the destruction of the financial system caused by men playing around with other people's lifetime savings. By which men specifically? Just a few thousand bankers, brokers, and financial players in New York, London, and a few other financial capitals. The answer: a law requiring all financial workers to submit themselves a one-hour lingam (or yoni) massage every morning, between 10 am and 11 am.

It is only after the traders and bankers have been drained of their hostility, excess sperm, and their immense lust for cash, corporations, shares, and countries that they will be permitted to show up for work. Landing up at their offices around noon, they may indulge in half an hour of good-humored trading or bank business before they head out for their 3-martini, tax-deductible lunches. Returning from lunch, at 3 pm, they do another hour of friendly trading and servicing the share accounts of senior citizens before they return home to be dutiful husbands and fathers.

Consider the savings:

From Banks and entire European countries that don't have to be bailed out: $2 trillion

From Wall Street firms that don't have to be bailed out: $2 trillion

From cuts in defense budgets worldwide: $2 trillion

Improved productivity from better education: $1 trillion

Reduced policing costs resulting from a big post-lingam fall in violent crime: $1 trillion

Imagine what the world could do with $8 trillion each year—imagine the jobs created, the roads, schools, and hospitals built, the medicines and antibiotics donated, the potential terrorists sent to good schools for less than the $200 million cost of the optional air-conditioning system, stereo, and leather seats on a $500 million B-1 bomber . . .

That's $8 trillion for a world population of 7 billion; even if half of it is used to improve infrastructure and give free medical care for everyone, the rest can be distributed to us common people, and it is still not something to sneeze at.

Not to sneeze at either is the great boost in Gross National Happiness and employment (all those new lingam specialist jobs, training institutes, and lingam massage parlors giving jobs to the construction industry), coupled with cuts in police forces, prison, and military spending . . . thus balancing national budgets all over the world.

Add to the above a lowered crime rate, a lower divorce and infidelity rate, and a kinder gentler humanity: it's nothing but win, win, win.

* * *

And now, to remedy this chapter's tilt towards lingams, I would like to devote the rest to yonis. Not only do I support Yoni massage for women's empowerment, I am all for it. You can't leave women out of any solution to the world's problems, and as women are increasingly better represented in many of the most important professions, any answer must fully recognize their importance.

The website of White Lotus East says: "Yoni is the Sanskrit word for the vagina that is loosely translated as 'sacred space' or 'Sacred Temple.' In Tantra, the yoni is seen from a perspective of love and respect. This is particularly important for men to learn."

I say: Amen. Count me in. I am an Eternal Worshipper at the said Temple, and my love and respect for the Yoni (or what E.L. James calls the Inner Goddess) is boundless as the Expanding Universe, which by the way is nothing but scientific jargon for the Cosmic Yoni. Not only do I volunteer my services (one free yoni massage a week, my gesture of giving back what the world of women has given to me), I urge inclusion of the Right to Yoni Massage as a sub-clause of the U.N. Charter's Universal Right to Massage.

But are they legal in most countries, including India? Unless they clearly are, I suggest including them in the Constitution. If they clearly are legal, I suspect that very soon, some enterprising businessman will soon start a chain of franchised establishments called *The Great Indian (or American)Pussy Rub,* which could become the Next Big Thing after Microsoft and Google.

Time for the Yoni Anti-Defamation League to take a strong stand and steamroller over all obstacles to yoni massage.

What about the Eastern Hemisphere? Despite the Filipino brouhaha over the rise of lingam massage in Cebu, my Filipino source, asked whether the Poor, Oppressed Yoni was getting its share, replied, "Not really."

What?! This is a grave injustice, one that we shall not take lying on our backs. There's no other alternative but for women's groups to march across the planet (a movement called Yonis Across The World, with the theme song from *And Justice for All Yonis* starring Gal Pacino?). For let us admit that the massage world, at least in the Eastern Hemisphere, tilts heavily towards lingams—and boy, since the Eastern Hemisphere also contains the overwhelming majority of the world's lingams, that is some tilt! If yoni massage were freely and widely offered, women would be more empowered and less easily enslaved; besides which, I am not only against wars fought with guns and bombs, but also the endless wars between the sexes, which rob humanity of so much of the energy we could devote to more crucial causes such as mosquito nets, cheap medicines, and better nutrition for Third World children, and of course, to global warming. Frequent yoni massages would leave us less inclined towards participating in such internecine wars.

How can such a massive change be achieved? Perhaps if the major powers of the world launched a Yoni Massage

Corps to serve the cause of women's empowerment in Third World countries, and also change United Nations Laws so that the International Court of Justice will, if necessary, hold world leaders down while they are being administered their compulsory lingam (or yoni) massages.

Imagine Shakespeare writing *Hamlet* in 2010. Instead of a speech starting with 'Poor Yorick!' it might have begun with: 'Poor Yoni!'

Or, to conclude with an ancient Sumerian poem, which reflects a timeless question and must always be a consideration in matters of social, national, international and interplanetary policy:

As for me, Inanna,
Who will plow my vulva?
Who will plow my high field?
Who will plow my wet ground?

Yes, indeed. So long as the world is blessed with vulvas, some three billion of them and rising at last count, someone or the other will have to plow them—or failing this onerous and crucial task (which ought to be added to the Millennium Development Goals), at least to massage them.

APPENDIX I: A MASSAGE CONSUMER'S WISH LIST

This section applies mainly to the United States and other Western countries, where massage costs around sixty dollars an hour, which is a sizeable chunk of a person's budget in these hard times; and in return for this expenditure, a massage customer ought to expect a certain standard of quality, professional competence, and humanistic treatment. Therefore, here, from my experience of over three thousand massages, is my tentative and humbly proposed bill of rights (which here is sometimes specific to men, but in many cases is unisexual).

Your masseuse ought to have reasonably soft hands, and clean and short fingernails; rough hands or long fingernails cause friction and end up giving the opposite of the soothing touch that one comes to a massage for.

With a masseuse you are experiencing for the first time, you have the right to leave in the first five minutes, without payment, or for a pro-rata payment for the time you were actually massaged.

You have the right to demand an active, hundred-percent hands on massage, without unsolicited New Age mumbo jumbo or spiritual interventions or administrations of any kind, unless it was advertised or listed as a New Age massage.

You have the right to a massage therapist who understands where the body parts are located, what their normal range of behavior is, and is not embarrassed or does not make you embarrassed about their existence, and is able to drape you efficiently without wasting more than 2 minutes of your time in the entire session so as to touch the maximum amount of skin with the exception of your actual sexual organ and your anus.

You have the right to be told about your massage therapist's years of experience and the school where he/she was qualified, and to have this fact prominently advertised on a signboard where you can see it.

You have the right to be given exactly the number of minutes of massage that you have paid for, and in no case less than 50 minutes when the massage is designated as a 1-hour massage. The massage therapist's questions or exploratory conversations, questionnaires, or draping ceremonies do not count towards the time of actual massage.

You have the right not to be suffocated by being excessively draped, and to demand that only the crucial portions of your anatomy be covered.

You have the right to a comfortable temperature in the place where you are massaged, and to a head rest that will not end up giving you worse neck cramps than when you started.

You have the right to your choice of oil or lotion, and to a reasonably *fresh* supply of the former.

You have the right to be touched, with real hands, and in every spot except your eyeballs, your penis, and on your various apertures. Once, a massage was going very badly (I had started faced down in a dark room), and I turned my head around, and discovered the masseuse was using a glove. I told her that touch was one of the most sacred contracts and justifications of a massage, and that I had felt violated by what she had done. She apologized, and took off her gloves.

Which leads me to the final point. The above bill of rights may not always be accepted, sometimes because a masseuse has received bad training or has come from a conservative way of thinking. Therefore, always try to be reasonable and explain your point of view, and be firm. I have often negotiated and ended up receiving a better massage through sheer persistence and sincerity.

Finally, the complicated thing about sex and sexual touch in massage, and men, is this: We want it, and we don't want it. We want it because we are human, and we don't want it because we may have another "significant other" in our lives at that very point, and we definitely don't want it if we are going to be tarred for it. If someone were to accept us for what we are, and do it, we wouldn't mind at all.

Further, here is a brief wish list that I and certain male (and possibly female) consumers may have in certain areas of massage. I realize that there may be some repetition in here, but the purpose is to emphasize a few important areas:

MARGINAL DIVERSITY OF RATES ABSURD

Why, in the U.S., does the worst massage costs forty-five dollars an hour, whereas the best massage, ten times as good, costs only seventy or eighty? In surgery, for example, the best surgeon may easily earn five times what the mediocre ones earn, and in sports the best athletes earn a thousand times better than mediocre ones, so why do the worst masseuses charge only 25 percent less than the best ones? An independent body ought to rate massage quality and suggest an appropriate fee, and masseuses should be required to display the rating, not just the certificate, so the customer can decide what quality he is getting for the money paid. So long as there are horrendously incompetent or uncaring practitioners charging fifty or sixty dollars an hour—which is a rip-off—the better ones will be able to charge much more, and far more than is fair. If a state body cannot do it, let an independent consumer body rate the masseuses, using questionnaires and anonymous testers, and publish the results on a web site.

CARING MAKES THE DIFFERENCE

To the few masseuses who regard massage as a purely mechanical job with cash coming in at the end of it: you have it wrong, because a masseuse is a care-giver. You must care. The best massage therapists, therefore, are those who, during the act of massage, are in a Mother-Child or Lover-Love-Object relationship with their client. Those who maintain a purely businesslike attitude in the massage room never give truly exceptional massages.

TOWEL/GLOVE MASSAGES

I don't mean masseuses who use towels to cover the subject's privates; I mean those who actually massage through a towel which is placed on the body of the subject, thus avoiding actual contact with the subject's skin! Or those who use gloves for the same purpose. Massaging through a towel or with gloves: it's like giving a handshake with a towel, or a hug with full body armor. Why even bother? Why not just make a namaste or a folded hands gesture as the Indians do and then ask the customer to buzz off, after having first collected your fee?

As for the glove massage, I remember when I was lying on the table face down in a dark room, and the masseuse entered and started massaging my back. Something about her touch felt wrong, so I turned over—and was shocked to notice the gloves, and felt outraged and violated. Why? I asked. For hygiene, she replied. But a massage is all about touch, I retorted—if not, why bother with this profession and why not become an accountant instead? To her credit, she apologized, and performed the rest of the massage without gloves.

So too the so-called New York State Draping Law: why don't these bureaucrats understand that all those prudish attempts to defeat sex don't defeat it; they simply make it more expensive?

NAILS AND ROUGH HANDS

In general, especially in the rougher, more tropical parts of the world where bacterial contamination could be a problem, I prefer that masseuses clip their nails completely, so as to avoid accidentally scratching my skin, and also to wash their hands with soap and water before a massage. However a few women do indeed know how to use their perfectly manicured long nails exquisitely to arouse and to titillate almost to a maddening point as a prelude to something much grander. These nails don't leave marks or incisions, and, when they choose, they are experts in strokes that use their fingers efficiently without having the nails dig into the skin. As this is a rare art, I generally ask to see a masseuse's hands before I agree to be massaged by her. In addition, as I am a writer and not a sumo wrestler, I often verify if her hands are soft; soft hands give me great pleasure, comfort, and reassurance; a rough hands massage, which may be the result of the masseuse having worked in the garden or done rough housework for long periods of time, feels abrasive and violating, like a sandpapering.

SHADY PLACES: AN INDICATOR
If you are asked to pay the money in advance, tell them it is the shady places that usually do that, and you were not looking for a shady place. Such places will pretend to "massage" you for about ten minutes, do a pretty shoddy job of it, and then ask you what you really want. If they still insist you pay in advance, and you don't want to risk losing your forty or sixty dollars, just walk out.

GOOD MASSEUSE ATTRIBUTES
What makes a good masseuse? In my experience it helps if he/she is happy, reasonably fulfilled, and at peace; and if they love cats, all the better. If your insides are full of turmoil, as happened with my long-term New York masseuse Janet, who was often in conflict with her mother and her boyfriends, you may have the world's best technique, yet end up infecting your customer with your disturbance and inner turmoil.

Above all, humility: a humility that regards every individual as unique, that respectfully asks the customer how the pressure suits them, and on how it is working for them, what special areas of pain they have. And after some initial small talk to put the customer at ease and to show human concern, silence is best, with phone calls and disturbances to be shunned except in emergencies.

RHYTHM AND MUSIC

One of the masseuses mentioned in this book, Noo No. 8, had this defect: her strokes had too many abrupt pauses, a one-minute spell of massage followed by a fifteen-second intermission, and again, and again, the rhythm being constantly interrupted like a car with dust in its carburetor or in its fuel. It is important to be rhythmic and orderly throughout the massage, so that the body isn't always guessing as to when and where the next stroke will land, and if possible to have harmonious, non-invasive, relaxing music playing in the background.

PHONE CALLS WHILE MASSAGING:

Janet's chief drawback was that she answered phone calls mid-massage from prospective customers responding to her two different advertisements, cradling her cordless telephone in one hand while massaging with just one hand where formerly she had used two. Soon I had memorized all her speeches, including her angry, irritated, or exasperated rejection of customers seeking happy endings or hand jobs, which she had recently taken off her menu.

I would never again repeat a masseuse who let this happen, because tranquility and total attention are crucial for a massage to work. Also, in the course of the phone calls, a masseuse's personal stresses are often passed on to the customer who may leave the studio well-massaged but still tense.

ABOUT THE AUTHOR

P.C. Anders or Peter Anders is a widely published author of more than twelve books of fiction, nonfiction, and humor, under other names. He is widely traveled New Yorker, who has lived in Asia for at least eight years. Taking a strong stand for freedom of expression, refusing to succumb to embarrassment or apology for realistic descriptions of the human body or natural functions, and blending humor with serious issues—these are a few of the features of his writing style. Among the writers who have influenced him, he credits Henry Miller, Mark Twain, Thomas Pynchon, Vladimir Nabokov, Joan Didion, Kurt Vonnegut, and Don De Lillo.

Peter is a passionate advocate of peace, humanism, and freedom of expression, and the author of four e-books: *Lingam Massage: A Safe Sex, Anti-War, and Economic Recovery Tool*, *The Uncensored Massage: Massage and Sex in America and Elsewhere*, *The Uncensored Massage: Thailand, Indonesia, Vietnam, and China,* and *The Uncensored Massage: Cambodia and the Czech Republic.* Please look for upcoming new books at amazon.com and other online portals. Also, he now publishes occasional blogs at uncensoredmassage.tumblr.com and has a Twitter feed: @imbooks.